Contents

Foreword   iv

Preface   v

Acknowledgements   vi

1 Causes of maternal deaths   1

2 Physiological and anatomical changes in pregnancy relevant
   to resuscitation   10

3 Resuscitation equipment   17

4 Principles of ECG monitoring   26

5 Basic life support   35

6 Advanced life support   54

7 Anaphylaxis   70

8 Records and record keeping   77

9 Reporting and managing a maternal death   81

10 Bereavement   88

11 Ethical and legal issues   92

12 Resuscitation training   101

Appendix   111

Bibliography   113

Index   119

Foreword

Normality is the basis for midwifery practice. Midwives are experts in the provision of care to mothers and babies who are progressing normally in the cycle of reproduction. It is therefore of utmost importance that when complications do occur that the midwife is able to recognize departure from the normal quickly, and to react immediately with knowledge and skill.

There is a saying in the Fire Service that the first five minutes of a fire are yours, the same principle applies to obstetric emergencies – the first five minutes are the midwife's. What the midwife does in that time-frame whilst awaiting medical aid may be the difference between mortality and morbidity.

Because the causes of obstetric shock may be different to collapse in other situations, it is essential to understand the underlying pathophysiology in order to initiate the appropriate treatment. As this book is concerned solely with pregnant and parturient women, it is directly relevant to midwives, and makes management of a life-threatening situation more likely to be successful. Guidelines for the management of obstetric shock and resuscitation of the mother based on the information in this book makes it a welcome addition to the body of knowledge which underpins good midwifery practice in both normal and abnormal situations.

Mrs N R Shaw
SRN, SCM, MTD, BA[Hons]
Midwife Assessor for England,
Confidential Enquiries into Maternal Deaths
Manager, Womens Services
Manor Hospital
Walsall

Preface

Cardiopulmonary arrest in pregnancy is uncommon, occurring once in every 30 000 late pregnancies. Unfortunately, survival from such an event is exceptional (Morris and Willis, 1999). In the event of a maternal cardiopulmonary arrest, a speedy, co-ordinated response is essential. Healthcare professionals should know what action to take in such a grave situation in order to promote positive outcomes for both the mother and the fetus. Although most of the standard resuscitation procedures can and should be applied, some will need to be modified because of the anatomical and physiological changes associated with pregnancy. In particular, aortocaval compression should be relieved and, if there is no response to initial resuscitation, a perimortem Caesarean section should be considered within 5 minutes of the arrest when there is fetal viability.

The aim of this book is to provide a comprehensive guide to resuscitation in pregnancy. It is hoped that the style of the book, together with the logical and systematic layout, will make the information readily accessible and easy to assimilate.

Philip Jevon
Margaret Raby

Acknowledgements

Why Mothers Die – Report on Confidential Enquiries into Maternal Deaths in the UK' Crown copyright material is reproduced with the permission of the Controller of Her Majesty's Stationary Office

The Report of the RCOG Working Party on Prophylaxis Against Thromboembolism in Gynaecology and Obstetrics has been reproduced with Permission from the Royal College of Obstetricians and Gynaecologists

Wendy Noble and West Midlands NHS Executive for reproducing 'Confidential Enquiries into maternal Deaths in the UK', West Midlands Region Guidance for Health Professionals (1997)

Resuscitation Council (UK) for the reproduction of their BLS, ALS and AED guidelines from the Advanced Life Support Manual (2000) and Resuscitation Guidelines 2000, and their BLS diagrams featured in 'Resuscitation for the Citizen'

ECGs reproduced with permission from Laerdal

The BMJ Publishing Group for the reproduction of their algorithm for the Emergency medical treatment of anaphylactic reactions

Nursing Times for the reproduction of their article by P. Jevon (2000)

Medical Photography Department for their help with the photographs

Chris Newson, Consultant Anaesthetist and midwives on the Delivery Suite, Manor Hospital Walsall for their help with the CPR photographs

Sharon Worth, RGN and Trainee Solicitor at Mills & Reeve in Birmingham, for her help with the Ethical and Legal Issues chapter

Janet Wheatley, Health Promotion Department, Walsall Health Authority for the BLS drawings

Chapter 1

Causes of maternal deaths

Introduction

Most maternal deaths result from acute pathology. An understanding of the causes of maternal deaths would therefore be helpful, as this provides an indication of the causes of cardiopulmonary arrest in pregnancy.

The aim of this chapter is to discuss the acute causes of maternal deaths, with particular reference to the most recent report on maternal mortality, *Why Mothers Die: Report on Confidential Enquiries into Maternal Deaths in the United Kingdom 1994–1996* (Department of Health, 1998) (Figure 1.1).

Objectives

By the end of the chapter the reader will be able to:

- classify a maternal death into one of four groups
- discuss the main causes of direct maternal deaths
- discuss the main causes of indirect maternal deaths
- state the main cause of fortuitous deaths
- state the main causes of late deaths.

Classification of maternal deaths

A maternal death is any death that occurs during or within 1 year of pregnancy, childbirth or abortion and is directly or indirectly related to these conditions. During the last triennium, 376 deaths were reported to

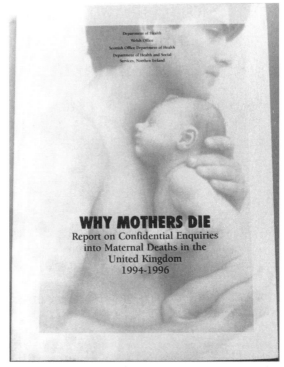

Figure 1.1 *Why Mothers Die: Report on Confidential Enquiries into Maternal Deaths in the United Kingdom 1994–1996* (DOH, 1998)

or identified by the enquiry (Figure 1.2). These deaths were classified into one of the following four groups:

1. Direct maternal death – death resulting from obstetric complications of the pregnant state (pregnancy, labour and puerperium) such as pulmonary embolism or amniotic fluid embolism, or from interventions, omissions, incorrect treatment, or a chain of events resulting from any of these.
2. Indirect maternal death – death resulting from a previous existing disease, or from a disease that developed during pregnancy that was not due to direct obstetric causes but was aggravated by the physiological effects of pregnancy (e.g. cardiac disease).
3. Fortuitous death – death resulting from unrelated causes that just happened to occur during pregnancy or puerperium (e.g. a road traffic accident).

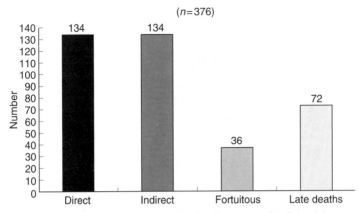

Figure 1.2 Classification of maternal deaths. *Report on Confidential Enquiries into Maternal Deaths in the United Kingdom 1994–1996* (DOH, 1998)

4. Late death – a death occurring between 42 days and 1 year following an abortion, miscarriage or delivery that is due to direct or indirect maternal causes.

Direct causes of maternal deaths

Figure 1.3 shows the direct causes of maternal deaths as reported to the enquiry (DOH, 1998).

Pulmonary embolism

Pulmonary embolism (PE) is still the major cause of maternal death in the United Kingdom. It accounted for 46 deaths, and these can be categorized as follows:

1. *Antepartum* – 18 deaths. Two-thirds occurred during the first trimester, including three following operative procedures.
2. *Postpartum* – 28 deaths.
   - Fifteen followed Caesarean section. Only a small proportion of these were in the > 35 years age group. Current guidelines recommend that women > 35 years should receive thromboprophylaxis, and the relatively low numbers of deaths in this age group might suggest that such treatment is effective.

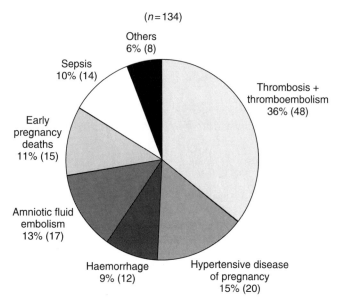

Figure 1.3 Direct causes of maternal deaths. *Report on Confidential Enquiries into Maternal Deaths in the United Kingdom 1994–1996* (DOH, 1998)

- Ten followed vaginal delivery. Of these, no deaths from PE occurred in the first week, and most occurred 2–4 weeks post-delivery.
- In three deaths the mode of delivery was unknown (the cause of death in these cases was ascertained from the death certificate, and the mode of delivery was not stated).

Some of the collapses and subsequent deaths occurred without warning and in the absence of apparent risk factors. However, in most cases the mothers had multiple risk factors or symptoms suggestive of PE and/or DVT. Risk factors include:

- obesity (booking weight > 80 kg)
- bed rest
- dehydration
- increasing age
- previous DVT and/or PE
- smoking.

Combination of risk factors, e.g. age and Caesarean section, can lead to an increase in risk greater than the additive effect of the two factors (Greer,

Table 1.1   Risk assessment profile for thromboembolism in Caesarean section

Low risk– early mobilization and hydration:

- Elective Caesarean section – uncomplicated pregnancy and no other risk factors

Moderate risk – consider one of a variety of prophylactic measures:

- Age > 35 years
- Obesity (> 80 kg)
- Para four or more
- Gross varicose veins
- Current infection
- Pre-eclampsia
- Immobility prior to surgery (> 4 days)
- Major current illness (e.g. heart or lung disease, cancer, inflammatory bowel disease, nephrotic syndrome)
- Emergency Caesarean section in labour

High risk – heparin prophylaxis ± leg stockings

- Patient with three or more moderate risk factors from above
- Extended major pelvic or abdominal surgery (e.g. Caesarean hysterectomy)
- A personal or family history of deep vein thrombosis, pulmonary embolism or thrombophilia; paralysis of lower limbs
- Patient with antiphospholipid antibody (cardiolipin antibody or lupus anticoagulant)

1997). It is hoped that the recommendations of the Royal College of Gynaecologists Working Party on Prophylaxis against Thromboembolism in Gynaecology and Obstetrics, 1995 (Table 1.1) will help to reduce the incidence of post-Caesarean section pulmonary embolism.

Pre-eclampsia and eclampsia

A total of 20 deaths were attributed directly to pre-eclampsia (12) and eclampsia (8).

- In eight other cases severe pre-eclampsia was a significant contributory factor, but the deaths were considered by the assessors to be directly due to other causes.

- The mean gestational age was 32 weeks (range 26–40).
- Fifty-five per cent of deaths were due to major deficiencies in care.

Cause of death

Acute Respiratory Distress Syndrome (ARDS) was the commonest cause of death. Other causes included:

- intracerebral haemorrhage
- subarachnoid haemorrhage
- pulmonary oedema
- pneumonia
- hepatic rupture
- hepatic failure.

Antepartum and postpartum haemorrhage

Twelve deaths were attributed to antepartum and postpartum haemorrhage; four to placental abruption, three to placenta praevia and five to postpartum haemorrhage.

Life-threatening haemorrhage occurs in 1 in 1000 pregnancies (Drife, 1997; Mantel *et al.*, 1998). Although the low number of deaths does suggest that in most cases treatment is effective, it must still be emphasized that death from obstetric haemorrhage can occur with frightening speed. The following must therefore be heeded:

- accurate estimation of blood loss
- prompt recognition and treatment of clotting disorders
- early involvement of a consultant haematologist
- involvement of a consultant anaesthetist in resuscitation
- use of adequately sized i.v. cannulae
- close monitoring of central venous pressure.

Amniotic fluid embolism

Seventeen deaths were caused by amniotic fluid embolism (AFE). It has a mortality rate of over 80 per cent (Morgan, 1979; Killam, 1985), and the risk increases with age.

- Only one woman was < 25 years of age, and the majority were > 30 years of age.
- The average childbearing age is rising, and this may be a possible cause of the rise in AFE.

- AFE is normally thought to be associated with labour induction and the use of oxytocic drugs. However, eight cases occurred prior to labour.
- Antenatal complications were present in 50 per cent of the cases (e.g. amniocentesis, polyhydramnios, placenta accreta, cervical suture, fibroids and intrauterine death).
- AFE occurred in only one entirely straightforward pregnancy.
- In nine cases, cardiac arrest followed the sudden collapse and resuscitation was impossible.

A UK Amniotic Fluid Embolism Register has been set up with the aim of identifying any common factors or differences between survivors and deaths. For further information and entry criteria, see Chapter 9.

Anaesthesia

Only one case was directly attributed to anaesthesia. In this case excessive doses of spinal anaesthetic were given together with large volumes of local anaesthetic injected into the epidural space, which caused extensive sympathetic block resulting in severe hypotension.

Indirect maternal deaths

Figure 1.4 shows the indirect causes of maternal deaths as reported to the enquiry (DOH, 1998).

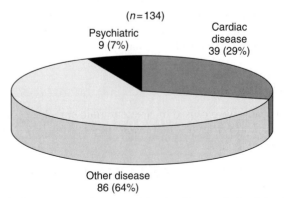

(n=134)

Psychiatric
9 (7%)

Cardiac
disease
39 (29%)

Other disease
86 (64%)

Figure 1.4 Indirect causes of maternal deaths. *Report on Confidential Enquiries into Maternal Deaths in the United Kingdom 1994–1996* (DOH, 1998)

Cardiac disease

Thirty-nine deaths were attributed to cardiac disease.

Congenital heart disease

Ten deaths were attributed to congenital heart disease:

- two to aortic valve disease complicated by endocarditis
- seven to pulmonary hypertension (ventricular septal defect, three; primary pulmonary hypertension, three; and hypertrophic obstructive cardiomyopathy, one)
- one to anomalous coronary arteries.

Acquired cardiac disease

Twenty-nine deaths were attributed to acquired cardiac disease:

- seven to aneurysm of the thoracic aorta and its branches
- four to puerperal cardiomyopathy
- four to cardiomyopathy and myocarditis
- six, all sudden and unexpected, to myocardial infarction
- eight to other causes.

Endocarditis is still a fatal complication of heart disease in pregnancy. In the last 12 years it has been the cause of 10 per cent of all cardiac-related deaths. Awareness of the possible risk, especially in mothers with a non-specific illness, is paramount.

Other diseases

There were 86 deaths from other diseases, including:

- nine from infectious diseases (e.g. pneumonia, toxoplasmosis)
- twelve from endocrine, metabolic and immunity disorders (e.g. phaeochromocytoma)
- forty-seven from central nervous system diseases (epilepsy accounted for 19 of these)
- six from circulatory system disorders (e.g. air embolism)
- seven from respiratory system disorders (e.g. asthma).

Psychiatric deaths

Nine women committed suicide, five during pregnancy and four within 6 weeks of delivery.

Fortuitous maternal deaths

Road traffic accidents were the leading cause of fortuitous deaths, 13 in total.

Late deaths

Seventy-two late deaths were reported:

- four were direct
- thirty-two were indirect, including 12 suicides
- thirty-six were fortuitous, four of which were cardiac related (three myocardial infarctions and one cardiac arrhythmia).

Summary

An outline of the acute causes of maternal deaths has been provided based on the findings of *Why Mothers Die: Report on Confidential Enquiries into Maternal Deaths in the United Kingdom 1994–1996* (DOH, 1998). An understanding of these causes will provide an indication to the causes of cardiopulmonary arrest in pregnancy.

Chapter 2

Physiological and anatomical changes in pregnancy relevant to resuscitation

Introduction

The physiological and anatomical changes in pregnancy can make the mother more susceptible to and less tolerant of cardiac arrest and its associated anoxic insults (Archer and Marx, 1974). In addition, they require modification of some of the standard resuscitation procedures. An understanding of these changes and the clinical implications for resuscitation is therefore essential.

The aim of this chapter is to outline the physiological and anatomical changes in pregnancy and discuss their relevance in resuscitation.

Objectives

By the end of this chapter the reader will be able to:

- discuss the relevant changes in the cardiovascular system
- discuss the relevant changes in the respiratory system
- discuss the relevant changes in the gastrointestinal system
- outline physiological fetal considerations.

Changes in the cardiovascular system

During pregnancy the maternal cardiovascular system undergoes a number of dramatic changes, which can be further influenced by gestational age, maternal position and labour (Figures 2.1, 2.2). Relevant changes are detailed below.

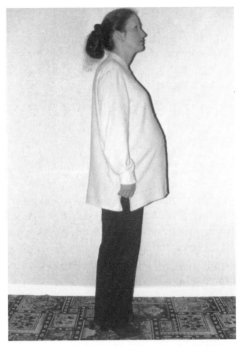

Figure 2.1 Physiological and anatomical changes in pregnancy relevant to resuscitation. *Cardiovascular changes* – heart rate ↑, cardiac output ↑, uteroplacental blood flow ↑; *Respiratory changes* – ventilation ↑ and partially compensated alkalosis, oxygen demand ↑, chest compliance ↓, functional residual capacity ↓; *Gastrointestinal changes* – slower gastric emptying, incompetent gastro-intestinal sphincter increases the risk of regurgitation of gastric contents

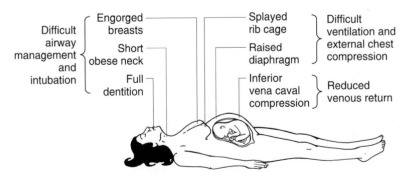

Figure 2.2 Specific difficulties with resuscitation in late pregnancy. Reproduced with kind permission from BMJ Publishing

Heart rate

The maternal heart rate will start to rise from as early as the seventh week of gestation. By late pregnancy it will have risen to approximately 20 per cent higher than the pre-pregnancy level (Lee and Cotton, 1991). Knowledge of this change is particularly helpful in the post-resuscitation period.

Cardiac output

During the first trimester, cardiac output begins to rise. By the end of the second trimester, it will have reached a peak approximately 40 per cent higher than in the pre-pregnancy period. The increases in heart rate and stroke volume both contribute equally to this rise (Clark *et al.*, 1989). This change is particularly significant because the need for an increased cardiac output will also be required during resuscitation. As a result, it is even more important to ensure that chest compressions are effective and any aortocaval compression is relieved.

Decrease in systemic vascular resistance and blood pressure

A decrease in the resistance in the pulmonary and uteroplacental circulations results in a reduction in systemic vascular resistance. This in turn will lead to a gradual lowering of mean arterial blood pressure during the first two trimesters, which only returns to pre-pregnancy levels by term (Sullivan and Ramanathan, 1985). Compared to pre-pregnancy, systolic and diastolic recordings can be 5–10 mmHg and 10–15 mmHg lower, respectively (Barron, 1984). Although a decrease in systemic vascular resistance and blood pressure is not significant during resuscitation, knowledge of the 'normal' blood pressure readings is important in the post-resuscitation period.

Uteroplacental blood flow

In a non-pregnant woman, the uterus receives less than 2 per cent of the total cardiac output (Lee *et al.*, 1986). However, during pregnancy the blood flow gradually increases until, at term, the uterus receives approximately 10 per cent of the cardiac output (Lee and Cotton, 1991). This blood flow is largely determined by maternal perfusion pressure (Doan-Wiggins, 1996). During resuscitation the uteroplacental blood flow will be markedly reduced because the maternal perfusion pressure will have dropped, and therapeutic doses of adrenaline administered to resuscitate the mother may in fact cause uteroplacental vasoconstriction, thus compromising the already diminished fetal blood flow (Lee *et al.*, 1986).

Aortocaval compression

During the second half of pregnancy, the weight and size of the gravid uterus can have profound effects on the maternal circulation. In the supine position, aortocaval compression can markedly effect blood flow in 90 per cent of women (Lee and Cotton, 1991). This compression will result in a fall in the venous return to the heart, leading to a reduction in the cardiac output by as much as 10–25 per cent (Kerr, 1965). In addition, pressure on the abdominal aorta can reduce arterial blood flow and increase venous pressure (Bieniarz *et al.*, 1968). This may lead to a reduced uteroplacental blood flow. In late pregnancy, aortocaval compression should be relieved (Figure 2.3).

Changes in the respiratory system

Increased oxygen consumption and basal metabolic rate

Maternal oxygen requirements increase by approximately 21 per cent (Lee and Cotton, 1991). At the same time, the basal metabolic rate rises by about 14 per cent (Archer and Marx, 1974). The net effect of these two changes is that the mother is more susceptible to hypoxia during cardiac arrest, and consequently early tracheal intubation and effective ventilation is required.

Hyperventilation and partially compensated respiratory alkalosis

Hyperventilation causes a state of partially compensated respiratory alkalosis. Consequently, during resuscitation the mother's buffering capacity is reduced and is therefore more susceptible to the effects of acidosis.

Decreased functional residual capacity

As pregnancy progresses, the pressure of the gravid uterus on the diaphragm increases. This results in a progressive fall in functional residual

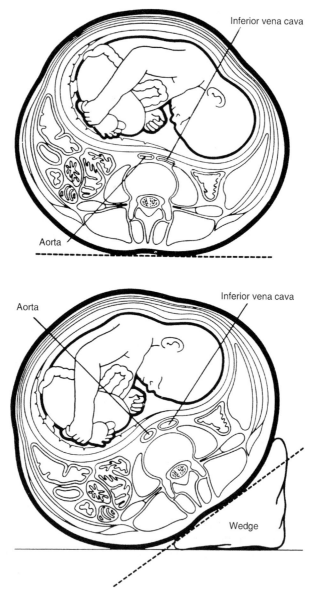

Figure 2.3 Aortocaval compression: relieved following lateral uterine displacement using a wedge. Reproduced from Churchill-Davidson, H. (1984). *A Practice of Anaesthesia*, published by Lloyd-Luke (Medical Books) Ltd, London. Original was reproduced courtesy of Gerald W. Ostheimer and Breon Laboratories, USA

capacity of the lungs. The mother is consequently more susceptible to hypoxia (Windle, 1968), and again resuscitation will be more difficult (Satin and Hankins, 1991).

Decreased chest compliance

Upward displacement of the diaphragm and viscera by the enlarging uterus will decrease chest compliance, and ventilation and chest compressions will therefore be more difficult (Lee *et al.*, 1986).

Changes in the gastrointestinal tract

There is a high risk of regurgitation of stomach contents leading to pulmonary aspiration in the arrest situation (Morris and Willis, 1999). Reasons for this include:

- reduced gastrointestinal motility resulting in slower gastric emptying (Doan-Wiggins, 1996)
- increased intragastric pressure
- an incompetent gastro-oesophageal sphincter.

Consequently, prompt airway management, cricoid pressure and early intubation by an experienced anaesthetist are essential in the management of a maternal arrest.

Physiological fetal considerations

Several physiological fetal adaptations and reflexes protect the fetus from the effects of maternal hypoxia. A beneficial redistribution of fetal blood occurs; selective peripheral vasoconstriction results in increased cerebral and myocardial blood flow (Seldon and Burke, 1988). In addition, there is greater oxygen saturation of fetal haemoglobin at any given partial pressure of oxygen. However, the vital organs can only be preserved for a limited time; if asphyxia persists, neurological damage or death will ensue. Unfortunately it is not possible to stipulate the length of time the fetus can survive because there are so many influencing variables, including effectiveness of resuscitation, stage of pregnancy and events leading up to the arrest (e.g. was the mother hypoxic?). There have been reported cases of infants surviving neurologically intact following delivery after more than 20 minutes of maternal resuscitation (Katz *et al.*, 1986). However this is a rare event, and current recommendations advocate emergency Caesarean section within 5 minutes of the arrest if the fetus is viable (European Resuscitation Council, 1998).

Summary

Anatomical and physiological changes in the cardiovascular, respiratory and gastrointestinal systems that accompany pregnancy can not only make resuscitation physically difficult, but also be deciding factors as to whether the mother and fetus survive. It is therefore important for practitioners to be aware of these changes so that they can modify their resuscitation techniques appropriately.

Chapter 3

Resuscitation equipment

Introduction

A speedy response is essential in the event of a cardiopulmonary arrest, and procedures should therefore be in place to ensure that all the essential equipment is immediately available, accessible and in good working order. A carefully set out and fully stocked cardiac arrest trolley is the ideal.

The aim of this chapter is to outline what resuscitation equipment should be available on the cardiac arrest trolley and make recommendations for the checking and maintenance of this equipment.

Objectives

By the end of this chapter the reader will be able to:

- describe a suggested layout for the cardiac arrest trolley
- discuss the procedure for routine checking of equipment
- discuss the procedure for checking equipment following a resuscitation
- discuss what equipment a community midwife should carry.

Layout of the cardiac arrest trolley

The cardiac arrest trolley (Figure 3.1) should be spacious, sturdy, easily accessible and mobile. All trolleys should be identically stocked to avoid confusion. Every Maternity Unit should compile an equipment inventory based on local requirements and circumstances (Figure 3.2).

It is most important to include only the bare essentials, as too much equipment can cause confusion and delay. Detailed below is a suggested layout for the trolley:

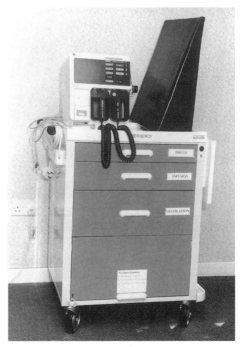

Figure 3.1   Cardiac arrest trolley

Top surface of trolley

- Defibrillator complete with ECG leads, electrodes and defibrillation pads
- Oxygen cylinder with flow meter, capable of delivering flow rates of 15 l/min, and oxygen tubing
- Wedge (Figure 3.3)
- Suction source, including suction tubing and catheters (this may be stored next to the trolley)
- Sharps box
- Dust sheet covering the trolley and the above equipment.

Drawer 1

Drugs:

- epinephrine/adrenaline 1 : 10 000 solution × 5
- epinephrine/adrenaline 1 : 1000 × 5

WALSALL HOSPITALS NHS TRUST
LAYOUT OF ADULT RESUSCITATION TROLLEY

TOP SURFACE DEFIBRILLATOR WITH LEADS + ELECTRODES ATTACHED   RUBBISH BAG ATTACHED
DEFIBRILLATION PADS   TO SIDE OF TROLLEY
                                                                        O2 Cylinder

FIRST DRAW - DRUGS MINI-I-JET DRUGS PACK

FOIL TRAYS WITH 20 ml SYRINGE x 2, 10 ml SYRINGE x 2, GREEN NEEDLES x 2, GREEN NEEDLES x 6, STERETS x 6

SECOND DRAW - INFUSION

IVI GIVING SET x 2		DISPOSABLE DRESSING TOWEL x 2 ECG/DEFIBRILLATION JEL
VYGON TROCAR CANNULA	MEDICUT CANNULA x 2	
TAGADERM/VECAFIX x 2	ECG PAPER	QUILLS x 2 SPINAL NEEDLES SIZE 16 g x 2 PULSATORS x 2
MICROPORE 1.25 cm + 2.5 cm	ELASTOPLAST 7.5 cm	
PAIR OF SCISSORS	VENFLON CAPS x 2	VENFLON 18 g(PINK) x 2 VENFLON 17 g(WHITE) x 2
	TWO WAY PLASTIC CONNECTOR	
ECG ELECTRODES x 6	CREPE BANDAGE 10 cm	VENFLON 20 g(GREEN)x 4

THIRD DRAW - VENTILATION

AMBU BAG, MASK (SIZES 4 + 5) WITH O2 RESERVOIR BAG + O2 TUBING   ET TUBES 6.5, 7, 8 + 9
SIZE 4 MASK   2 LARYNGOSCOPES (ONE LARGE BLADE & ONE SMALL)
GUEDEL AIRWAYS - SIZE 2, 3 + 4   CATHETER MOUNT
GAUZE AND KY JELLY   WHITE COTTON TAPE ROLL
SPARE BATTERIES + BULBS FOR LARYNGOSCOPE   10 ml SYRINGE
ARTERY FORCEPS   ENDOTRACHEAL TUBE INTRODUCER

BOTTOM SHELF

MULTIPLUG SOCKET ADAPTER   SUCTION TUBING
NON-STERILE GLOVES   YANKEURS SUCKERS x 2
SHARPS BOX   GREEN SUCTION CATHETERS x 4
TROLLEY SEAL   JUNE 1998

Figure 3.2 Resuscitation equipment inventory – a suggested layout

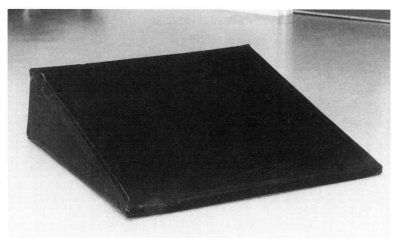

Figure 3.3   Wedge

- atropine 1 mg/10 ml × 3
- lidocaine/lignocaine 2%/10 ml × 1
- calcium chloride 10% × 1
- naloxone 400 µg/ml × 1
- amiodarone 300 mg
- sodium chloride 0.9% 10 ml × 5
- sodium chloride 0.9% 500 ml × 2
- i.v. fluids, e.g. haemacel × 2
- selection of syringes/needles (wherever possible use pre-filled syringes (Figure 3.4) rather than ampoules).

Drawer 2

Equipment for intravenous access and infusion:

- selection of wide-bore cannulae and preferred securing device
- i.v. tubing
- air inlet set
- tape
- bandage
- pressure bag × 2
- scissors
- three-way tap
- cannula caps.

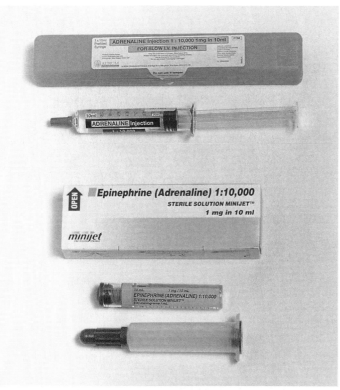

Figure 3.4 Pre-filled syringes

Drawer 3

Airway/ventilation equipment:

- Guedal airways, sizes 2, 3 and 4
- self-inflating bag fitted with oxygen reservoir bag and oxygen tubing
- masks, sizes 4 and 5
- laryngoscopes × 2, with size 3 and 4 Macintosh blades
- spare batteries and laryngoscope bulbs
- cuffed tracheal tubes sizes 7, 8 and 9
- 10-ml syringe
- bougie
- tracheal tube introducer
- lubricating gel

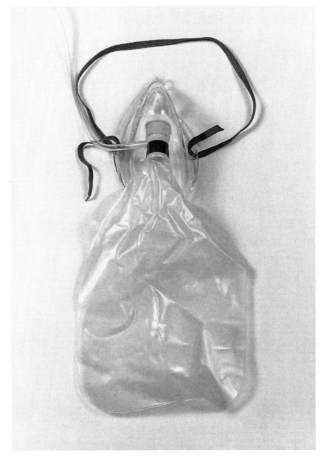

Figure 3.5 Oxygen mask with non-rebreathe bag

- oxygen mask with non-rebreathe bag (Figure 3.5)
- laryngeal mask and combitube in the event of failed intubation.

Bottom shelf

- Gloves, aprons and eye shields/visor
- Suction tubing/catheters
- Spare defibrillation pads
- Spare ECG electrodes stored in airtight packaging
- Extension lead/multiplug adaptor.

Routine daily checking of equipment

A system for daily documented checks of the equipment inventory should be in place. Some cardiac arrest trolleys can be 'locked' with a numbered seal (Figure 3.6) after being checked. Once the contents have been checked, the trolley can then be sealed and the seal number documented by the person who has checked the trolley. The advantage of this system is that an unbroken seal, together with the same seal number last recorded, signifies the trolley has not been opened since it was last checked and sealed. The equipment inventory should therefore be complete. A broken seal or an unrecorded seal number suggests the inventory may not be complete, hence a complete check is required. The seal can easily be broken if the trolley needs to be opened.

Expiry dates should be checked (drugs, fluids, ECG electrodes, defibrillation pads etc.). Laryngoscopes, including batteries and bulbs, should also be checked to ensure that they are in good working order. The self-inflating bag should be checked, following manufacturer's recommendations, to ensure that there are no leaks and that the rim of the facemask is adequately inflated.

The defibrillator should be checked on a daily basis following the manufacturer's recommendations. This usually will involve charging up

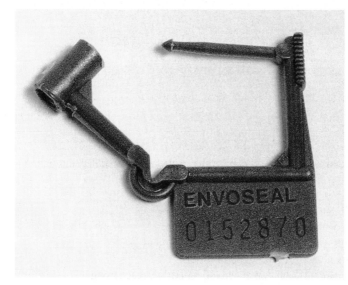

Figure 3.6 Trolley seal

and discharging the shock into the defibrillator. It is recommended that advice is sought from a member of the Electrobiomedical Engineers' Department (EBME) or from the manufacturer's representative regarding how to do this. In addition, most defibrillators need to be plugged into the mains to ensure that the battery is fully charged in the event of use. ECG electrodes attached to the defibrillator leads should be checked to ensure that the gel is moist; if they are dry, they should be replaced.

All mechanical equipment (e.g. defibrillator, suction machine) should be inspected and serviced on a regular basis by the EBME Department following the manufacturer's recommendations.

Checking of equipment following use

Restocking after a resuscitation procedure should be a specifically delegated responsibility. As well as the routine checks identified above, any disposable equipment used should be replaced and re-usable equipment (e.g. self-inflating bag) cleaned following local infection control policies and manufacturer's recommendations. Any difficulties with equipment encountered during resuscitation should be documented and reported to the relevant personnel.

Equipment for community midwives

Community midwives should carry basic resuscitation equipment. What this includes will depend on individual circumstances and level of training. A suggested list of equipment includes:

- airways
- a protective barrier for mouth-to-mouth ventilation
- a pocket mask
- a self-inflating bag
- a hand-held suction device
- an oxygen cylinder, oxygen tubing and an oxygen mask.

It is ideal to have all the equipment together in a handy carrying bag (Figure 3.7).

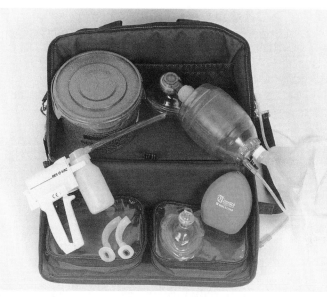

Figure 3.7 Community midwife's resuscitation bag

Summary

This chapter has detailed what resuscitation equipment should be immediately available in the event of a maternal arrest. Suggestions have been made regarding layout, storage, checking and maintenance of this equipment.

Chapter 4

Principles of ECG monitoring

Introduction

ECG monitoring forms an integral part of resuscitation. Once the presenting rhythm of the electrocardiogram (ECG) has been identified, any appropriate treatment can then be administered. However, poor technique can easily lead to an inaccurate ECG trace and mistaken diagnosis. An understanding of the principles of ECG monitoring is therefore essential.

The aim of this chapter is to outline the principles of ECG monitoring. In addition, basic ECG rhythms and life-threatening arrhythmias will be described.

Objectives

By the end of this chapter the reader will be able to:

- describe the conduction system of the heart
- describe the ECG and its relation to cardiac contraction
- outline the principles of ECG monitoring
- recognize sinus rhythm, sinus tachycardia and sinus bradycardia
- recognize life-threatening arrhythmias.

The conduction system of the heart

The heart possesses specialized muscle cells that initiate and conduct electrical impulses, resulting in myocardial contraction. This conduction system (Figure 4.1) comprises the following:

- sinus node (sinoatrial or SA node)
- atrioventricular node (AV node or AV junction)

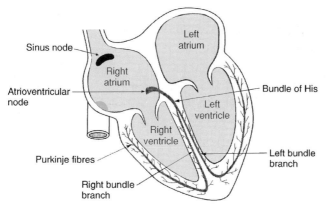

Figure 4.1 The conduction system of the heart

- bundle of His
- bundle branches (right and left)
- Purkinje fibres.

Nervous control of the heart rate

The sinus node normally acts as the pacemaker for myocardial contraction, and the rate at which it fires is dependent upon the autonomic nervous system:

- An increase in parasympathetic activity slows down the heart rate, while a decrease results in a faster heart rate. Atropine blocks the vagus or parasympathetic nerve, causing an increase in heart rate.
- The sympathetic nerve prepares the body for 'fight and flight', resulting in an increase in heart rate and in the force of myocardial contraction. Betablockers shield the heart from sympathetic nerve stimulation, resulting in a fall in heart rate and blood pressure and a reduction in myocardial workload.

The ECG and its relation to cardiac contraction
(Figure 4.2)

1. The sinus node fires and the electrical impulse spreads across the atria, causing atrial contraction (P wave).

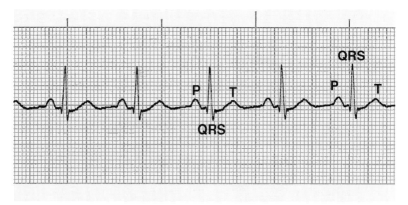

Figure 4.2 The PQRST complex

2. On arriving at the AV node, the impulse is delayed to allow the atria time to contract fully and eject blood into the ventricles. This brief period of absent electrical activity is represented on the ECG by a straight (isoelectric) line between the end of the P wave and the beginning of the QRS complex.
3. The impulse is then conducted to the ventricles through the bundle of His, right and left bundle branches and Purkinje fibres, causing ventricular depolarization and contraction (QRS complex).
4. The ventricles then repolarize (T wave).

Monitoring the ECG

Common characteristics of defibrillators and cardiac monitors

Regardless of whether a cardiac monitor or a defibrillator is used for monitoring the ECG, both generally have the following characteristics:

- A screen for displaying the ECG trace (some have a dull/bright mode switch which should be adjusted if the ECG trace and background is too dark).
- An ECG printout facility (particularly useful for recording arrhythmias); this documented evidence is invaluable both for prescribing treatment and also for the maternal records
- A heart rate counter, which calculates the heart rate by counting successive QRS complexes. However if the complexes are too small

they may not be counted, and in addition it can mistake large T waves and muscle movement for QRS complexes, again resulting in inaccurate heart rate readings. When relying on the heart rate counter, the practitioner should be aware of these limitations. To minimize or avoid this problem, the securing of an accurate ECG trace is necessary.

- Monitor alarms, which sound if the heart rate falls outside pre-set limits. These are not set during resuscitation, but are invaluable in the post-resuscitation phase when close monitoring will be required. However, if they are used and relied upon they must be set within agreed and safe parameters.
- A lead select switch – lead 2 is usually the best lead for ECG monitoring (**NB:** occasionally the defibrillator paddles are placed on the chest to secure an ECG trace, in which case the 'paddles' switch should be selected on the defibrillator. If the 'paddles' switch is selected but ECG leads are used, a straight line and no ECG trace will result).

Establishing an accurate ECG trace

A suggested method for establishing an accurate ECG trace is as follows:

1. Switch the defibrillator/monitor on.
2. Attach the ECG electrodes. The recommended ECG electrode position, which benefits from reduced muscle interference and will not hinder CPR or defibrillation, is as follows:
   - red on the right shoulder
   - yellow on the left shoulder
   - green on the left lower abdominal wall.
3. Select lead 2 on the defibrillator/monitor.
4. Briefly stop chest compressions while the ECG is interpreted.
5. If a straight line is seen, check the gain (ECG size) on the monitor, check all the connections, and check that lead 2 has been selected.

Difficulties encountered with ECG monitoring

Numerous problems can be encountered during ECG monitoring, some due to the limitations of the monitoring system itself and others to improper technique. Detailed below are common problems encountered, including measures on how to avoid them. This information is particularly useful in the post-resuscitation period.

ECG electrodes

The ECG electrodes should be in date, with the gel sponge moist (not dry). If there are difficulties in obtaining a clear ECG trace, wiping the skin with an alcohol wipe may help. If the patient is sweating profusely, a small amount of tincture benzoin applied to the skin and then left to dry before the application of the electrodes is an option (Jowett and Thompson, 1995). Although this technique is not really practical in a cardiac arrest situation, it is perhaps worth considering in other situations.

Wandering baseline

The height of the QRS complexes may vary with the mother's position and respiration. This may also cause a wandering baseline (i.e. the ECG trace going up and down). If this problem persists, the electrode position should be changed or a different monitoring lead selected.

Interference and artefacts

Poor electrode contact, patient movement and electrical interference (e.g. from infusion pumps by the bed) can cause a 'fuzzy' appearance on the ECG trace. Efforts should be made to minimize interference and ensure that the electrode contact is secure and reliable.

Sinus rhythm, sinus bradycardia and sinus tachycardia

Sinus rhythm

Sinus rhythm (Figure 4.3) is the normal rhythm of the heart. The impulse originates in the sinus node at a rate of 60–100 beats/min, is regular, conducted down the normal pathways, and is conducted with no abnormal delays.

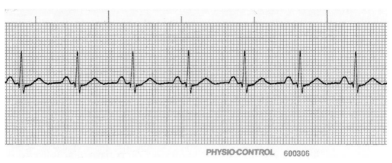

PHYSIO-CONTROL 600306

Figure 4.3 Sinus rhythm

NB: Sometimes sinus rhythm without a pulse (electromechanical dissociation) can be seen during a cardiac arrest.

Sinus tachycardia

- The ECG shows the same characteristics as sinus rhythm except that the ventricular rate is > 100 beats/min (Figure 4.4).
- Causes include drugs (e.g. hydralazine, rotodrine), pyrexia, acute blood loss, anxiety and pregnancy.
- If treatment is required, it is normally directed at the primary cause.

Sinus bradycardia

- The ECG shows the same characteristics as sinus rhythm except that the ventricular rate is < 60 beats/min (Figure 4.5).
- Causes include vagal stimulation, increased intracranial pressure, drugs (e.g. betablockers), hypothermia and severe pain.

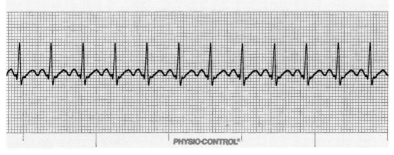

Figure 4.4 Sinus tachycardia

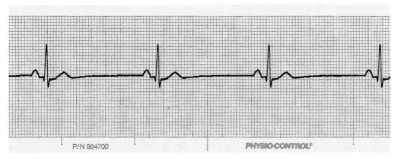

Figure 4.5 Sinus bradycardia

- Treatment will depend on the situation. If the mother is symptomatic, administer atropine 500 µg i.v.; repeat if necessary. Oxygen should also be administered.

Cardiac arrest arrhythmias

Ventricular fibrillation

Ventricular fibrillation (Figure 4.6) is where all co-ordination of electrical activity in the ventricular myocardium is lost, resulting in cardiopulmonary arrest.

- The ECG is characteristic, showing a bizarre irregular waveform which is apparently random in both amplitude and frequency. It can be classified as either coarse or fine. Certainly the latter is significant in the resuscitation situation because it can be mistaken for asystole, particularly if there is some interference.
- The definitive treatment is rapid defibrillation.

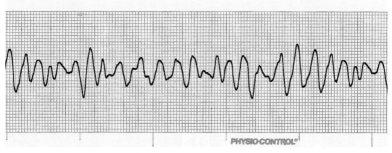

Figure 4.6 Ventricular fibrillation

Ventricular tachycardia

Ventricular tachycardia (Figure 4.7) usually results from a focus in the ventricles firing at a rapid rate. The mother may or may not lose cardiac output.

- The ECG shows a rapid heart rate, usually over 150 beats/min, and the QRS complex is characteristically wide (> 2.5 small squares). The ECG configuration can vary depending on where in the ventricles the focus is.
- If it causes a cardiopulmonary arrest, the definitive treatment is rapid defibrillation.

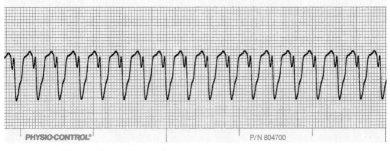

Figure 4.7 Ventricular tachycardia

Asystole

- Although asystole (Figure 4.8) is often referred to as a 'straight line', in reality in the early stages it is usually an undulating line.
- In all cases of apparent asystole, the ECG trace should be viewed with suspicion before arrival at a final diagnosis. Other causes of a straight-line ECG trace should be excluded (e.g. incorrect lead setting, disconnected leads and ECG gain too low). It is important not to miss ventricular fibrillation.

Electromechanical dissociation or pulseless electrical activity

Electromechanical dissociation (EMD) or pulseless electrical activity is when the mother has had a cardiopulmonary arrest, but the ECG trace appears normal (e.g. sinus rhythm, Figure 4.3). The diagnosis is made from

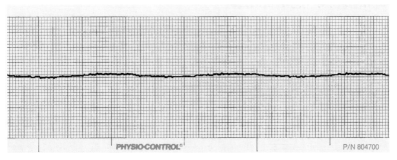

Figure 4.8 Asystole

a combination of the clinical absence of a cardiac output together with an ECG trace that would normally be associated with a good pulse.

EMD may be present in severe obstetric haemorrhage that has resulted in a loss of cardiac output.

Summary

Monitoring the ECG is essential both during resuscitation and in the post-resuscitation period. This chapter has identified how best the ECG can be monitored, including how to avoid the common pitfalls. In addition, basic rhythms and life threatening arrhythmias have been described.

Chapter 5

Basic life support

Introduction

The most critical period in the management of a maternal cardiopulmonary arrest is the first few minutes of the event (Dildy and Clarke, 1995). In the non-pregnant woman, failure of the circulation for 3–4 minutes will usually lead to irreversible cerebral damage. In pregnancy, the physiological and anatomical changes render the mother more susceptible to hypoxia during periods of apnoea (Archer and Marx, 1974). A speedy response is therefore essential in the event of a maternal cardiopulmonary arrest.

Once respiratory or cardiac arrest has been diagnosed, the mother should be positioned appropriately and basic life support (BLS) started immediately. The purpose of BLS is to maintain adequate ventilation and circulation. It is often only a holding procedure, buying time while the means of reversing the underlying cause of the arrest can be obtained or a Caesarean section (if required) performed.

The term BLS refers to maintaining an open airway and supporting breathing and circulation without the use of equipment other than a protective shield. For practical purposes, this chapter will also cover the use of basic resuscitation equipment.

The aim of this chapter is to understand how to perform effective BLS following current guidelines (Resuscitation Council, UK, 2000).

Objectives

By the end of the chapter the reader will be able to:

- discuss the initial assessment and state the sequence of intervention in BLS

- outline the basic principles of airway management
- describe three methods of ventilation
- describe how to apply cricoid pressure
- describe the correct procedure for chest compressions
- outline the management of choking.

Initial assessment and sequence of intervention in BLS

The procedures described below and the sequence in which they are carried out are based on Resuscitation Council, UK (2000) recommendations. When more than one healthcare professional is present some of the actions described will be undertaken simultaneously.

On seeing a mother collapse or on finding a mother who is apparently unconscious call out for help/pull the emergency buzzer (ensure the environment is safe before approaching – this is unlikely to be a problem in the hospital setting, but outside potential hazards could include traffic and toxic fumes).

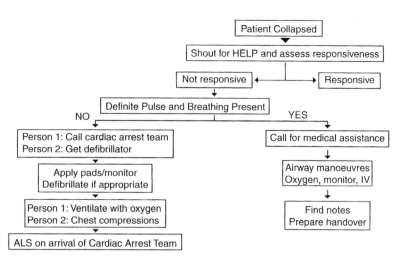

Figure 5.1 Resuscitation Council (UK) Basic Life Support Algorithm (2000)

Assess responsiveness. Gently shake the mother's shoulders and ask her loudly "are you alright?" If she responds try and establish the likely cause of the collapse and get help if necessary. If there is no response proceed to checking breathing and circulation.

Assess breathing, pulse and signs of circulation. Open the airway by tilting the head and lifting the chin (use jaw thrust if trauma to the neck is suspected). Ensure the airway is clear and check for signs of breathing for no longer than 10 seconds; look for chest movements, listen for airflow at the mouth and nose and feel for airflow on your cheek.

While checking for breathing, feel for a carotid pulse. As it can sometimes be difficult to determine the presence of a carotid pulse (Flesche et al., 1994; Eberle et al., 1996; Bahr et al., 1997), also assess for other signs of circulation (e.g. patient movement, swallowing).

If the mother is breathing, monitor her vital signs and the fetal heart (Cox and Grady, 1999) and ensure medical help is on the way. Administer oxygen, commence ECG monitoring and secure intravenous access following local protocols.

If the mother is not breathing or there is no pulse, ensure the cardiac arrest team, anaesthetist, obstetrician and paediatrician are alerted, again following local protocols. Also summon/fetch CPR equipment, including the defibrillator. If outside hospital, ensure the paramedics and if appropriate the Obstetric Flying Squad are alerted.

Start resuscitation. Ventilate with oxygen and start chest compressions if there is no pulse, at a rate of 100 per minute (ratio of two ventilations:15 compressions). Once the defibrillator arrives apply ECG leads/defibrillation pads. If indicated defibrillation should be performed as soon as possible by a practitioner trained to do so.

NB: In the third trimester, the inclined left lateral position should be adopted as soon as possible (Skinner and Vincent, 1993). Cricoid pressure should be applied if staff numbers allow.

When to get help

When more than one person is present, one can start resuscitation while the other gets help. However, the practitioner is faced with a dilemma if he or she is alone. The decision will be influenced by local protocols and the availability of emergency medical services. In most situations it would be advisable to get help before starting resuscitation; however, if the cause of the collapse is likely to be related to drowning, trauma, drugs or alcohol intoxication prompt resuscitation for 1 minute may actually revive the mother and should precede activation of the emergency services (Resuscitation Council, UK, 2000).

Basic principles of airway management
Head tilt/chin lift

The head tilt/chin lift manoeuvre (Figure 5.2) is considered the most effective method of opening the airway in an unconscious patient (Idris *et al.*, 1996), achieving airway patency in 91 per cent of situations (Guildner, 1976). By stretching the anterior tissues of the neck, it will displace the tongue forward away from the posterior pharyngeal wall and lift the epiglottis from the laryngeal opening (Safar, 1958). A pillow under the head may help to maintain this position. In the presence of a possible cervical spine injury, e.g. following a road traffic accident, the jaw thrust is a safer option.

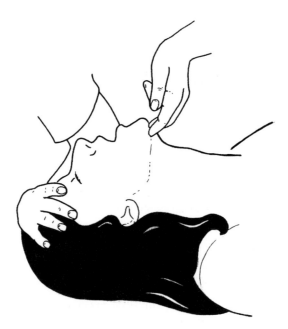

Figure 5.2   Head tilt and chin lift manoeuvre to open the airway

Jaw thrust

An alternative method is the jaw thrust manoeuvre. The mandible is displaced anteriorly (together with the tongue) using the index fingers positioned just proximal to the angles of the jaw. At the same time, pressure by the thumbs on the chin helps to open the mouth. The jaw thrust is favoured in trauma, as head tilt could aggravate a cervical spine injury.

Dentures

The mother is unlikely to have dentures. However, if she does, leave well-fitting ones in place because they can help to maintain the normal shape of the face. This will help the practitioner to achieve a better seal when ventilating.

Suction

The airway should be cleared of any vomit, secretions etc. A rigid wide-bore (Yankaeur) catheter (Figure 5.3) can provide rapid suction of large

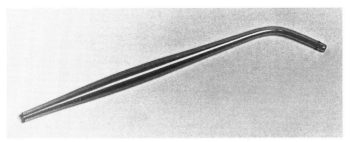

Figure 5.3 Rigid wide-bore (Yankaeur) catheter

volumes of fluid from the mouth and pharynx. A flexible catheter is useful for suctioning down an oropharyngeal airway and a tracheal tube. In order to minimize deoxygenation, suction should last no longer than 10 seconds at a time (Idris *et al.*, 1996).

Oropharyngeal airway

The oropharyngeal airway (Guedel airway; Figure 5.4) is a useful airway adjunct. It is relatively easy to insert, and can provide an artificial passage to airflow by separating the posterior pharyngeal wall from the tongue.

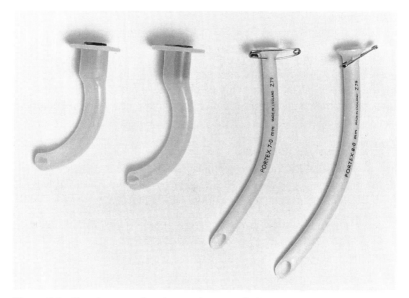

Figure 5.4 Oropharyngeal and nasopharyngeal airways

Cautions

The oropharyngeal airway should only be used in the unconscious mother, as it may induce vomiting and laryngospasm (Mehta, 1990). The correct size should always be estimated, and the correct insertion technique will help to minimize complications.

An appropriate-sized airway is one that holds the tongue in the normal anatomical position and follows its natural curvature (Idris *et al.*, 1996). The correct size can be estimated by placing the airway against the face and measuring it from the mother's incisors to the angle of the jaw (Resuscitation Council, UK, 2000). A variety of different sizes are available, though a size 2 or 3 is normally adequate for most women.

It is important to select the correct size. If it is too big, it may actually block the airway, hinder the use of a facemask and damage laryngeal structures. If it is too small, it may block the airway by pushing the tongue back.

Procedure for insertion

In order to avoid unnecessary trauma to the delicate tissues in the mouth and inadvertently blocking the airway, the following procedure for insertion is recommended:

1. If possible, lubricate the airway.
2. Insert it into the mouth in the inverted position and, as it passes over the soft palate, rotate it through 180.° The curved part of the airway will help depress the tongue and prevent it from being pushed posteriorly during insertion.
3. Following insertion, check and regularly monitor the position and patency of the airway and continue to maintain head tilt/chin lift.

Nasopharyngeal airway

The nasopharyngeal airway (Figure 5.4) is made from soft plastic with a flange at one end and a bevelled edge at the other. It is less likely to induce gagging than an oropharyngeal airway, and it can be used in a semiconscious or conscious mother when the airway is at risk of being compromised (e.g. sometimes in the post-resuscitation phase). It can be life saving in a mother with a clenched jaw, trismus or maxillofacial injuries. It is contraindicated if there is a suspected base of skull fracture, as it may penetrate the cranial fossa (Muzzi *et al.*, 1991).

It is important to determine the correct sized airway. If it is too small it will not be effective, and if it is too long it may enter the oesophagus (causing distension and hypoventilation) or stimulate the laryngeal or glossopharyngeal reflexes (causing laryngospasm and vomiting). The tubes are sized in millimetres according to their internal diameter, and the larger the diameter, the longer the length. Adult sizes range from 6–8 mm, and the correct size is comparable to the size of the mother's little finger (European Resuscitation Council, 1998).

Procedure for insertion
1. Where appropriate, explain the procedure to the mother.
2. Check the right nostril for patency.
3. Insert a safety pin through the flange. This is a precautionary measure to prevent inhalation of the airway.
4. Lubricate the airway.
5. Insert the airway into the nostril, bevelled end first. Pass it vertically along the floor of the nose, using a slight twisting action, into the posterior pharynx (if there is resistance, remove the airway and try the left nostril). Once inserted, the flange, which should be at the level of the nostril, can be taped in place.
6. Reassess the airway and check for patency and adequacy of ventilation. Continue to maintain correct alignment of the airway and chin lift as necessary, and constantly reassess patency.

The laryngeal mask airway

The laryngeal mask airway (LMA) is a curved, wide-bore tube with an inflatable cuff at the distal end which is designed to seal the hypopharynx around the laryngeal opening, leaving the tube orifice close to the opening of the glottis. It enables the establishment of a clear airway and can facilitate ventilation.

Although the LMA is commonly used in the resuscitation of non-pregnant patients, its use in maternal resuscitation has yet to be evaluated. Unfortunately it does not protect the airway from aspiration of gastric contents; an uncommon problem in non-pregnant patients (Owens *et al.*, 1995), but a major concern and certainly a high risk in maternal resuscitation. At present probably the only place for the LMA in maternal resuscitation is in the event of a failed intubation. However, this may change, and for completeness the procedure for insertion is described in the Appendix.

Three methods of ventilation

The most common cause of failure to ventilate is improper positioning of the head and chin (Idris *et al.*, 1996).

Mouth-to-mouth ventilation

The procedure for mouth-to-mouth ventilation is as follows:

1. Position the mother correctly; supine in early pregnancy and left lateral tilt in late pregnancy.
2. While maintaining head tilt and chin lift, pinch the soft part of the nose using the index finger and thumb of the hand holding the mother's forehead.
3. Open the mother's mouth, maintain chin lift and take a breath in (Figure 5.5).
4. Place your lips around the mother's mouth, ensuring there is a good seal.
5. Blow steadily into the mother's mouth over about 2 seconds, watching for chest rise. Avoid high tidal volumes and the associated high airway pressures as these may lead to gastric inflation and regurgitation, particularly if cricoid pressure has not been applied. Tidal volumes as low as 400–600 ml are adequate to make the chest rise (Baskett *et al.*, 1996).

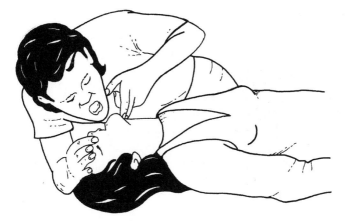

Figure 5.5 Open the mother's mouth, maintain chin lift and take a deep breath in

6. While still maintaining head tilt and chin lift, remove your mouth and watch for the mother's chest to fall as the air comes out.
7. Repeat the above sequence.
8. If there is no chest movement following ventilation, check that the airway is open and there is an adequate seal, and remove any obstruction from the mouth. Allow up to five attempts to achieve two effective ventilations; if still unsuccessful, move on to assess for signs of circulation.

Mouth-to-mask ventilation (pocket mask)

A well-fitting pocket mask (Figure 5.6) used by a trained practitioner is an effective method of ventilation. Common characteristics of the pocket mask are that it is transparent in design, thus enabling prompt detection of any vomit or blood in the airway; it has a nipple for the attachment of supplementary oxygen; and it has a one-way valve directing the mother's expired air away from the rescuer.

The procedure for mouth-to-mask ventilation is as follows:

1. Position the mother correctly; supine in early pregnancy and left lateral tilt in late pregnancy.
2. If available, attach an oxygen source to the nipple at a flow rate of 10 l/min. This will allow the delivery of up to 50 per cent oxygen (Lawrence and Sivaneswaran, 1985).

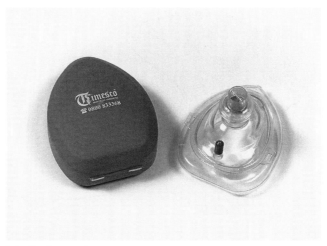

Figure 5.6 Pocket mask

3. Press the mask against the patient's face and lift the chin into it by applying pressure behind the angles of the jaw; also tilt the head.
4. Ventilate steadily over 2 seconds, watching for chest rise. Avoid high tidal volumes and the associated high airway pressures as these may lead to gastric inflation and regurgitation, particularly if cricoid pressure has not been applied. Tidal volumes as low as 400–600 ml are adequate to make the chest rise (Baskett *et al.*, 1996).
5. While still maintaining head tilt and chin lift, watch for the mother's chest to fall as the air comes out.
6. Repeat the above sequence.
7. If there is no chest movement following ventilation, check that the airway is open and there is an adequate seal with the mask, and remove any obstruction from the mouth. Allow up to five attempts to achieve two effective ventilations; if still unsuccessful move on to assess for signs of circulation.

Bag/valve/mask ventilation

Although the bag/valve/mask (Figure 5.7) device allows the delivery of higher concentrations of oxygen, the method requires considerable skill and may in fact be ineffective when undertaken by one person (Harrison and Maull, 1982; Hess and Baran, 1985). Consequently, a two-person technique is recommended (Hess and Baran, 1985; Jesudian *et al.*, 1985);

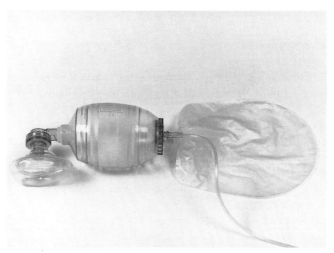

Figure 5.7 Bag/valve/mask device

one person to open the airway and ensure a good seal with the mask while the other squeezes the bag (Figure 5.8). An oxygen reservoir bag should ideally be used, as this will enable the delivery of higher concentrations of oxygen.

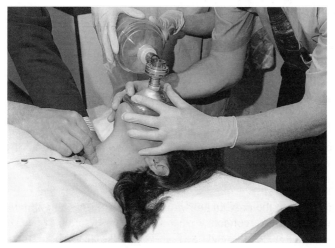

Figure 5.8 Bag/valve/mask ventilation: the two-person technique

The procedure for bag/valve/mask ventilation is as follows:

1. Position the mother correctly; supine in early pregnancy and left lateral tilt in late pregnancy.
2. Connect oxygen to the bag/valve/mask device at a flow rate of at least 10 l/min (follow the manufacturer's recommendations). This will usually achieve an inspired oxygen concentration of approximately 90 per cent.
3. Select an appropriate size mask. The mask should comfortably cover the mouth and nose, and should not cover the eyes or override the chin. It should be transparent, thus enabling prompt detection of any vomit or blood in the mouth, and should have a soft pliable edge to facilitate achieving a good seal.
4. Press the mask against the face and lift the chin into it by applying pressure behind the angles of the jaw; also tilt the head.
5. Ask a colleague to ventilate steadily over 1.5–2 seconds, watching for chest rise (squeeze the self-inflating bag, not the oxygen reservoir bag). Avoid high tidal volumes and the associated high airway pressures as these may lead to gastric inflation and regurgitation, particularly if cricoid pressure has not been applied. Tidal volumes as low as 400–600 ml are adequate to make the chest rise.
6. While still maintaining head tilt and chin lift, watch for chest fall.
7. Repeat the above sequence.
8. If there is no chest movement following ventilation, check that the airway is open and there is an adequate seal with the mask, and remove any obstruction from the mouth. Allow up to five attempts to achieve two effective ventilations; if still unsuccessful, move on to assess for signs of circulation.

Volume and rate of ventilation

Unless the mother's airway is secured with a cuffed tracheal tube, ventilation carries a high risk of gastric inflation, regurgitation of gastric contents and pulmonary aspiration (Melker, 1985). This risk of gastric distension is dependent upon:

- pressure in the proximal airway, which is influenced by inflation rate and ventilatory volume
- head and neck alignment and patency of the airway
- the opening pressure of the lower oesophageal sphincter.

To minimize the risk of gastric inflation, the following recommendations are made:

- Give slow ventilations over 2 seconds
- Use small ventilation volumes, just sufficient to achieve visible chest rise – 400–600 ml is adequate for ventilation because carbon dioxide production during a cardiac arrest is very low (Baskett *et al.*, 1996)
- Ensure a patent airway
- Apply cricoid pressure.

Cricoid pressure

Cricoid pressure was first introduced by Sellick (1961), who advocated its use during the induction of anaesthesia to reduce the incidence of aspiration of gastric contents. More recently, it has been recommended for use during resuscitation (Melker and Banner, 1985), particularly in late pregnancy, until the airway is protected by a cuffed tracheal tube (Morris and Willis, 1999).

The high incidence of pulmonary aspiration during cardiac arrests (Lawes and Baskett, 1987) emphasizes the need for all practitioners to be aware of the value of cricoid pressure during maternal resuscitation, and to be competent and safe at administering it.

Mode of action

If administered correctly, cricoid pressure will occlude the lumen of the oesophagus. This will have a two-fold effect; it will help prevent regurgitation and aspiration of gastric contents, and also inflation of the stomach.

Technique (Figure 5.9)

1. Locate the cricoid cartilage – the first complete ring of cartilage below the thyroid cartilage (the Adam's apple).
2. Place the index finger and thumb on either side of the cricoid cartilage.
3. Apply backward pressure to obstruct the lumen of the oesophagus, which is lying posteriorly; counterpressure may also be applied at the back of the neck, but this is not recommended if a neck injury is suspected.

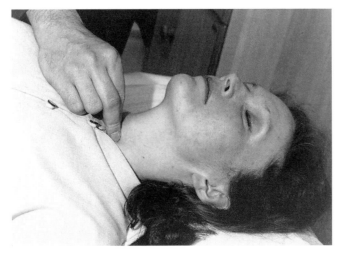

Figure 5.9 Cricoid pressure

4. Only release the pressure when the airway is protected by a cuffed tracheal tube (i.e. when the anaesthetist says so) or if the mother actively vomits.

Cautions

Cricoid pressure should not be applied during active vomiting because there is a risk of laceration to the oesophagus (European Resuscitation Council, 1998).

The anatomy of the airway can be distorted if too much pressure is applied, and this could hinder tracheal intubation.

Chest compressions

Position of the mother

The mother will need to be placed on a firm, flat surface. In early pregnancy (< 24 weeks) the mother can be left supine, but during the latter half of pregnancy, autocaval compression and decreased venous return in the supine position must be minimized by displacing the gravid uterus (Doan-Wiggins, 1996). There are four methods of achieving this:

- using pillows or a wedge
- using the Cardiff resuscitation wedge

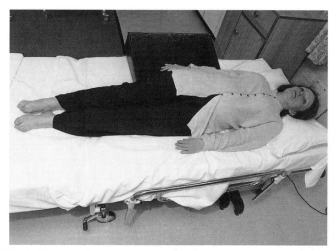

Figure 5.10 Left lateral tilt for chest compressions

- using a human wedge
- manually displacing the uterus.

Whichever method is used, it is most important that the displacement of the gravid uterus, or the lateral tilt, is over to the left and not to the right.

Using pillows or a wedge
Placing pillows or a wedge (Figure 5.10) under the mother's right side and hip provides a quick and probably the most practical method of displacing the gravid uterus in a maternal arrest in the hospital environment.

Using the Cardiff resuscitation wedge
The Cardiff resuscitation wedge is designed to be portable, yet sufficiently substantial to withstand CPR. It is made of plywood and is laminated with plastic for easy cleaning. The positioning of the mother allows easy access for procedures, and it is also possible to position the mother with pillows to facilitate intubation. Its use for resuscitation has been favourably evaluated (Rees and Willis, 1988).

Using a human wedge
An alternative method is to use a human wedge (Goodwin and Pearce, 1992). This is where one person kneels on the floor, sitting on his or her heels. The mother is then positioned so that her back is leaning against the

thighs of the person kneeling on the floor (the 'human wedge'). The 'human wedge' then stabilizes the mother's shoulders with one hand and the pelvis with the other. The head can be supported with a pillow or a rolled up item of clothing. Although this method of relieving aortacaval pressure can be employed anywhere by anyone, it should perhaps only be considered when a wedge or pillows are not available because it ties up a valuable member of the team.

Manually displacing the uterus

If no wedge is available, manual displacement of the uterus to the left and towards the mother's head is an acceptable alternative (Morris and Willis, 1999). However, this technique involves expertise and occupies a valuable member of the team.

Procedure for chest compressions

1. Locate the lower half of the sternum. Using the index and middle fingers, identify the lower rib margins and slide up them to the xiphisternum (where the sternum meets the ribs). Place the middle finger on this point and position the index finger on the sternum. (Figure 5.11).
2. Slide the heel of the other hand down the sternum until it reaches the index finger. Leave the heel of the hand here and place the other hand on top. Interlock the fingers and lift them up to ensure that pressure is not exerted on the mother's ribs (Figure 5.12). Correct positioning is

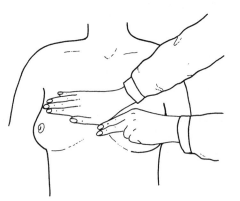

Figure 5.11 Chest compressions – locate the xiphisternum, place the middle finger on this point and position the index finger on the sternum, then slide the heel of the other hand down to meet the index finger

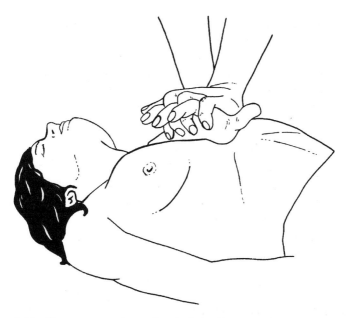

Figure 5.12 Chest compressions – interlock the fingers

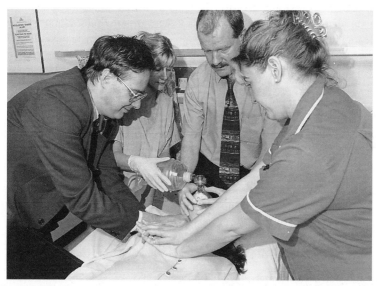

Figure 5.13 Chest compressions in late pregnancy – displaced gravid uterus

essential, as multiple liver lacerations can result from protracted chest compressions (Lau, 1994).

3. With arms straight and at right angles to the mother's chest, begin chest compressions (Figure 5.13).
4. Compress the chest approximately 4–5 cm, at a rate of 100 compressions per minute. It is important to release to allow ventricular filling. Compression and release times should be the same, as this will help to maximize arterial pressures (Taylor *et al.*, 1977). The pressure should be firm and controlled, and not erratic.
5. Combine chest compressions with ventilations at a ratio of 15:2. A pause of chest compressions is required for ventilations (once the patient is intubated the pause is not required. Deliver ventilations at a rate of approximately 12 per minute).

In early pregnancy, the standard position for chest compressions should be adopted.

Management of choking

Complete obstruction of the airway by a foreign body is a life-threatening emergency, and is often characterized by a sudden inability to talk, maximal respiratory efforts and the development of cyanosis. In addition, the mother may clutch her neck. When there is partial airway obstruction, the mother will be distressed and coughing and there may be an associated wheeze. If there is complete airway obstruction the mother will be unable to speak, breathe or cough, and she will eventually lose consciousness.

Treatment

If the mother is choking but still breathing, encourage her to cough. If she shows signs of becoming weak or stops breathing or coughing:

1. Call out for help.
2. Remove any obvious foreign body from the mouth, including any loose dentures. Support the mother's chest with one hand, lean her well forward and deliver up to five sharp slaps between her shoulder blades using the heel of the hand. (If the mother has collapsed, roll her onto her left side, support her chest with your thigh and then deliver the back slaps).

In the non-pregnant patient, abdominal thrusts are recommended at this stage. However, if the mother becomes unconscious chest compressions may be required to relieve the obstruction (Resuscitation Council, UK, 2000) as abdominal thrusts would be both difficult to deliver and potentially hazardous to both the mother and the fetus.

Summary

Prompt and effective BLS is an essential in the event of a maternal arrest. It buys time until the means can be obtained to reverse the underlying cause of the arrest, or until a Caesarean section can be performed. This chapter has discussed the sequence of BLS and described its main components in detail.

Chapter 6

Advanced life support

Introduction

Advanced life support (ALS) is the term used to describe the more specialized techniques employed to support breathing and circulation during resuscitation, as well as specific treatment used to try and restore cardiac output. The delivery of ALS should be in accordance with Resuscitation Council, UK, guidelines (2000).

The ALS algorithm (Figure 6.1) is universally applicable, though specific modifications are required to maximize the likelihood of success in a maternal arrest. When a cardiac arrest occurs before the onset of fetal viability, which is about the twenty-fourth week of gestation, the objectives of ALS are directed almost entirely at reviving the mother (Doan-Wiggins, 1996). In this situation, fetal survival depends very much on the successful resuscitation of the mother. However, beyond the twenty-fourth week of gestation the life of the potentially viable fetus must also be considered (Lee *et al.*, 1986).

The aim of this chapter is to provide an overview of ALS in maternal resuscitation based on current recommendations from the Resuscitation Council UK (2000).

Objectives

By the end of the chapter the reader will be able to:

- outline the ALS algorithm
- discuss the principles of defibrillation
- discuss the principles of tracheal intubation
- describe the recommended routes for drug delivery
- list the common drugs used in resuscitation
- discuss the role of Caesarean section in resuscitation
- describe the priorities in post-resuscitation care.

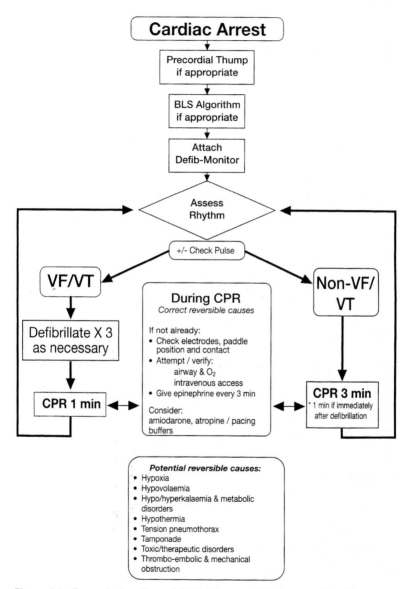

Figure 6.1 Resuscitation Council (UK) Advanced Life Support Algorithm

The ALS algorithm

Background to the algorithm

The commonest primary arrhythmia at the onset of a cardiac arrest in adults is ventricular fibrillation (Figure 6.2), or pulseless ventricular tachycardia (Sedgwick *et al.*, 1994). It is an eminently treatable rhythm, with most eventual survivors of a cardiac arrest belonging to this group (Tunstall-Pedoe *et al.*, 1992). Rapid defibrillation is the definitive treatment; the chances of success decline substantially with each passing minute (Cobbe *et al.*, 1991).

The ALS algorithm therefore focuses on the importance of quickly establishing an accurate ECG trace and determining whether defibrillation is required or not. This priority is equally important in maternal arrests, even though the incidence of ventricular fibrillation is probably lower than in the non-pregnant patients.

Using the algorithm

As in other areas of medical practice, guidelines must be interpreted with common sense and with an appreciation of their intent. The limitations of the algorithm must be recognized.

Entry into the algorithm depends on the events surrounding the cardiac arrest. If BLS is already in progress, then this should continue while the monitor/defibrillator is attached. ECG monitoring provides the link between BLS and ALS. If the patient is already monitored, clinical and ECG detection of cardiac arrest will be almost simultaneous. The presenting cardiac arrest rhythm can then be classified into one of two groups, dependent upon whether defibrillation is required or not, and the appropriate pathway is then followed. Each step that follows in the algorithm assumes that the previous one has been unsuccessful. Looping the algorithm reinforces the concept of constant reassessment. Each of the two pathways (VF/VT and non-VF/VT) will now be discussed.

VF/VT pathway

If the mother is in ventricular fibrillation, or pulseless ventricular tachycardia (VF/VT), rapid defibrillation is required. The recommended initial energy sequence for defibrillatory shocks is:

- 200 J
- 200 J
- 360 J.

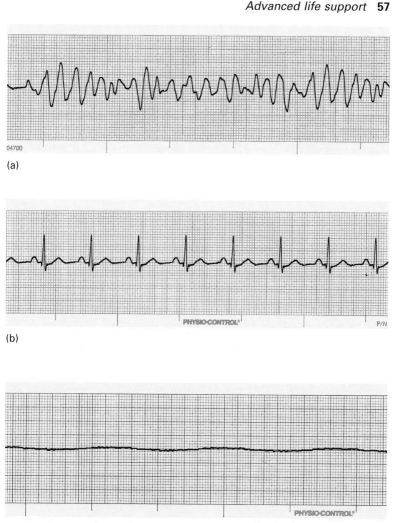

04700

(a)

PHYSIO-CONTROL

P/N

(b)

PHYSIO-CONTROL

(c)

Figure 6.2 Ventricular fibrillation (a), electromechanical dissociation (b) and asystole (c)

If the first 200 J shock fails, the second 200 J shock may be successful if delivered promptly because of reduced tissue impedance. Subsequent shocks should be at 360 J. After each shock, the ECG is reassessed to ascertain whether further defibrillation is required. Pulse checks following defibrillation are only recommended if an ECG compatible with a cardiac output is produced, or if there is uncertainty regarding accurate inter-pretation of the ECG. BLS should not interrupt the sequence of shocks unless there are undue delays with defibrillation.

Over 80 per cent of patients who are successfully resuscitated will be defibrillated by one of the first three shocks (Cobbe *et al.*, 1991). However, if these fail the priority changes to the provision of basic life support for 1 minute to help preserve cerebral and myocardial function (ideally during this period tracheal intubation and intravenous access should be secured and epinephrine/adrenaline administered). The ECG trace is then reassessed and further shocks of 360 J, again in groups of three, delivered if indicated. Each loop of the algorithm provides a further opportunity, if not already achieved, to secure intravenous access and tracheal intubation.

In persistent VF/VT, aggravating factors (e.g. drug toxicity) should be identified and if possible corrected. Although there is no convincing evidence to advocate their use, an anti-arrhythmic drug such as lig-nocaine may be considered after three to four loops of the algorithm. At this stage it is worth trying an alternative defibrillation position (e.g. anterior/posterior paddle placement) and also another defibrillator.

Non-VF/VT

If VF/VT can be positively excluded, defibrillation is not indicated at this stage and the non-VF/VT pathway of the algorithm is followed. The main arrhythmias normally seen are either pulseless electrical activity (PEA) or asystole (Figure 6.2). It must be stressed that VF can be mistaken for asystole if:

- the ECG leads become disconnected
- the gain (ECG size) is too low
- there is movement artefact
- the defibrillator/monitor is incorrectly set or is malfunctioning.

Great care should therefore be taken to ensure that the ECG trace is accurate. In asystole and PEA if there is bradycardia, as well as adrenaline, atropine 3 mg should be administered once only. After three minutes of CPR, the ECG trace should be reassessed and the appropriate pathway followed.

NB: Asystole immediately following defibrillation is common. In this situation continue CPR for 1 minute and then reassess the ECG trace as either VF or indeed sinus rhythm with cardiac output may have ensued. Adrenaline and atropine should be withheld during this minute.

Principles of defibrillation

Defibrillation is the untimed (asynchronous) depolarization of a critical mass of the myocardium to allow spontaneous sinoatrial node activity to resume. There is no contraindication to defibrillation in pregnancy, and there are reported cases of it being used without adverse effects on the fetus (Curry and Quintana, 1970; Stokes *et al.*, 1984). The defibrillator is shown in Figure 6.3.

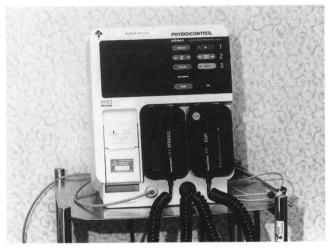

Figure 6.3   Defibrillator

Successful defibrillation requires the passage of sufficient electrical current to the heart. This current flow depends on the energy delivered (joules) and the transthoracic impedance (i.e. resistance to current flow). Factors influencing transthoracic impedance include:

- paddle pressure – 10 kg per paddle is recommended (Resuscitation Council, 2000)
- paddle–skin contact – gel pads should be used to improve conduction; bare paddles will result in high chest impedance (Sirna *et al.*, 1988; Figure 6.4)
- time interval between shocks – a short time interval between shocks will help to reduce impedance
- chest size
- phase of respiration.

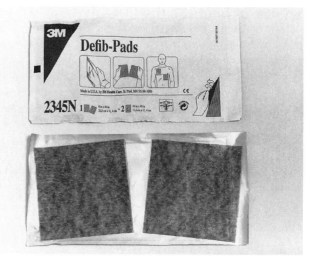

Figure 6.4 Defibrillation gel pads

Paddle position

One paddle is placed just to the right of the sternum below the right clavicle and one over the apex, avoiding the breast tissue (Pagan-Carlo *et al.*, 1996). The paddles are often labelled 'sternum' and 'apex'. Placing the paddles according to their namesakes is only important when monitoring through them or when undertaking cardioversion. For defibrillation it is not important (Resuscitation Council, UK, 2000).

Safety issues

There are a number of safety issues related to defibrillation. In particular, direct and indirect contact with the mother should be avoided – all personnel should be well away from the bed and not touching the mother or anything attached to the mother/bed (e.g. i.v. infusion stands, i.v. infusions etc.). The use of gel pads will minimize the risk of skin burns (and improve conduction), and any open oxygen source should be temporarily removed from the mother.

Automated external defibrillators (AED)

Operating a manual defibrillator requires extensive training and knowledge. Its use has therefore been traditionally restricted to doctors and to senior nurses working in critical care areas. However, modern automated external defibrillators abolish the need for the operator to have ECG interpretation skills and instructions are provided on screen or by voice prompts (or both).

As less operator training is required, they can be used by a wider range of personnel. Although automatic defibrillators are becoming increasingly common on the general wards, their deployment in Maternity Units is not thought to be prevalent. However, there is certainly a place for automated defibrillators in maternity care, and their use is now being included in authoritative texts (Cox and Grady, 1999). This is an area of clinical practice that needs to be evaluated. The Resuscitation Council (UK) algorithm for automated external defibrillation is therefore shown here for completeness (Figure 6.5).

Interventions during resuscitation

During maternal resuscitation it is important to:

- relieve aortocaval pressure and perform effective BLS using 100 per cent oxygen
- check and regularly re-check the ECG trace, ensuring that it is accurate and reliable
- defibrillate if indicated
- intubate as soon as possible (apply cricoid pressure until the airway is secured by a cuffed tracheal tube)
- establish two routes of i.v. access using wide-bore cannulae, and administer a fluid bolus
- administer adrenaline 1 mg every 3 minutes
- externally pace if required
- administer other drugs if indicated
- identify and treat any potentially reversible causes of the arrest
- if indicated, perform Caesarean section.

Potentially reversible causes of maternal arrest

The search for, and treatment of, any potentially reversible cause of the maternal arrest is paramount. Potentially reversible causes of cardiopulmonary arrest can conveniently be classified into two groups for ease of memory; four 'Hs' and four 'Ts' (Resuscitation Council, UK, 2000).

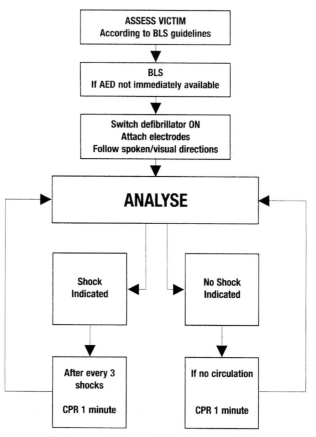

Figure 6.5 Algorithm for the use of automated external defibrillators.
Resuscitation Council (UK) Algorithm for Automated External Defibrillation

Hypoxia

The mother should be intubated and ventilated with 100 per cent oxygen.

Hypovolaemia

If the mother is haemorrhaging, intravascular volume should be restored with appropriate fluids. Urgent surgery to stop the bleeding may be required.

Hyperkalaemia/hypokalaemia and metabolic disorders

Electrolyte and metabolic disorders will probably only come to light following laboratory tests. However, the patient's history (e.g. renal failure) may be suggestive of an abnormal blood chemistry.

Hypothermia

Hypothermia should be suspected following an immersion injury. A low reading thermometer should be used, and efforts to rewarm the mother must be started (e.g. infusion of warm i.v. fluids).

Tension pneumothorax

Possible causes of tension pneumothorax include trauma and asthma. It could also complicate central venous cannulation. Immediate life-saving treatment is needle thoracocentesis (through the second intercostal space on the mid-clavicular line of the affected side) followed by insertion of a chest drain.

Tamponade

Cardiac tamponade occurs when blood or other fluid fills the pericardial space, raising intrapericardial pressure, compressing the heart and preventing it from filling (Nolan and Gwinnett, 1998). The clinical signs of cardiac tamponade include distended neck veins, hypotension and muffled heart sounds. Unfortunately, these can be obscured by the arrest itself. The history and clinical examination may be helpful, and it should be suspected in chest trauma. Initial treatment is needle pericardiocentesis to relieve the tamponade.

Thromboembolic or mechanical obstruction pulmonary embolism and amniotic fluid embolism

Amniotic fluid embolism is rare, but has 80 per cent mortality (Killam, 1985). The substitution of packed red cells, platelets, fresh frozen plasma and other blood derivatives may be necessary (Bussen *et al.*, 1997). Successful resuscitation following an amniotic fluid embolism has been reported (Hwang *et al.*, 1993). An emergency hysterectomy may need to be performed if the bleeding cannot be stemmed, and could be life saving (Leitner *et al.*, 1995).

Pulmonary embolism is more common. An emergency pulmonary embolectomy is the definitive treatment (Lau, 1994), and can be life saving (Ilsaas *et al.*, 1998). If possible, the mother should be transferred to a cardiovascular surgical department.

Streptokinase may also be useful in thrombolysis if these facilities are not immediately available.

Toxic/therapeutic disturbances

Magnesium sulphate is being increasingly used for the treatment and prevention of eclampsia. An accidental overdose of magnesium can cause cardiac arrest. In this situation, the administration of calcium gluconate 10% has been successful (Swartjes *et al.*, 1992) and should therefore be considered (Morris and Willis, 1999).

Cardiac arrest following epidural anaesthesia for Caesarean section has been reported (Myint *et al.*, 1992). Cardiac arrhythmias due to bupivacaine toxicity are probably best treated with bretylium and cardioversion rather than lignocaine (Morris and Willis, 1999).

Tracheal intubation

Tracheal intubation with a cuffed tube is the best method of securing the upper airway, and should be performed as soon as possible. It enables suction of the trachea and lower airways and delivery of high concentrations of inspired oxygen, and facilitates mechanical ventilation. The risks of gastric distension, regurgitation and aspiration of gastric contents, which are not uncommon during BLS, are minimized.

Intubating a pregnant woman can be difficult and potentially hazardous, particularly during a resuscitation situation, and it is therefore essential that an experienced anaesthetist is involved at an early stage. Describing the procedure for intubation is beyond the scope of this book. However, knowledge of the equipment required by the anaesthetist is helpful. A suggested list of equipment includes:

- MacIntosh curved blade laryngoscope×2, in working order
- tracheal tubes 7.0–8.0 mm (internal diameter)
- suction source
- oxygen source
- 10-ml syringe
- catheter mount
- tape to secure the tube
- gum elastic bougie and stylet
- bag/valve/mask device
- stethoscope.

Ineffective ventilation following intubation

Ventilation may not be established effectively after intubation, or may become ineffective after a variable period. The main causes of this can be described by the acronym DOPE:

- *D*isplaced tube (e.g. into the pharynx, oesophagus, right or left main bronchus)
- *O*bstructed tube (e.g. by vomit, blood, secretions etc.)
- *P*neumothorax
- *E*quipment failure.

These problems should be recognized and diagnosed by the checks that routinely follow intubation.

Drug delivery routes

Venous

The venous route remains the optimum method of drug administration during resuscitation. Venous access, using a wide-bore cannula, needs to be established as quickly as possible. The chosen access will depend on the circumstances and expertise available.

The peripheral route is least invasive, has minimal complications and does not interfere with CPR. However, drugs can take 1–2 minutes to reach the central circulation (Khun *et al.*, 1981). Following drug administration, a 20-ml bolus of 0.9% normal saline and elevation of the limb are therefore recommended (Emerman *et al.*, 1990). A second line should be secured if possible.

The central route (e.g. subclavian or internal jugular) can provide higher drug concentrations and has minimal circulation time. Unfortunately, it is more difficult to establish and can interrupt resuscitation, and complications can be catastrophic (Table 6.1).

Endobronchial

Both clinical and experimental studies have reported conflicting evidence about the efficacy of the endobronchial route for drug administration. It is therefore only recommended as a second-line approach. Adrenaline/epinephrine, atropine and lignocaine/lidocaine can be administered via this route (NB: not calcium or sodium bicarbonate).

Doses of two to three times the standard i.v. dose diluted up to a total volume of at least 10 ml of 0.9% normal saline is currently advocated

Table 6.1 **Complications of central venous cannulation**

- Arterial puncture
- Haematoma
- Haemothorax
- Pneumothorax
- Air embolism
- Damage to surrounding structures
- Arrhythmias
- Sepsis

(Aitkenhead, 1991; Hapnes and Robertson, 1992). This should then be injected beyond the tip of the tracheal tube and, to ensure dispersal to the distal bronchial tree and maximize absorption, should be followed by five ventilations. The rate of absorption will depend on the efficiency of the resuscitation, and will be reduced in the presence of pulmonary oedema.

Intracardiac

Intracardiac injection (i.e. injection directly into the ventricles) is no longer recommended (Resuscitation Council, UK, 2000) because it can be difficult to perform, may interrupt resuscitation, and carries a high risk of complications (e.g. laceration of the coronary artery).

Drugs commonly used in resuscitation
Adrenaline (epinephrine)

Adrenaline is routinely administered during resuscitation, as it improves coronary and cerebral blood flow in the mother (Michael *et al.*, 1984). Unfortunately it may induce uteroplacental vasoconstriction, particularly when maternal hypoxaemia or hypotension is present.

The dose is 1 mg (10 ml of 1 : 10 000 solution) i.v. repeated every 3 minutes. If the tracheal route is used the dose is 2–3 mg (2–3 ml of 1 : 1000 solution).

Atropine

Atropine antagonizes the action of the vagus nerve, and is administered when there is symptomatic bradycardia or asystole. The suggested dose for symptomatic bradycardia is 500 µg i.v. (repeated doses can be given). In asystole or EMD associated with a bradycardia, the maximum dose of 3 mg i.v. is administered once only (Resuscitation Council, UK, 2000); if the tracheal route is used, 6 mg in a volume not exceeding 20 ml may be given.

Anti-arrhythmic drugs

There is little evidence to support the use of anti-arrhythmic drugs during a cardiac arrest. However their use should be considered when defibrillation fails to terminate ventricular fibrillation or pulseless ventricular tachycardia. Amiodarone is the first drug of choice. Lignocaine (lidocaine) is an alternative if amiodarone is not available.

Calcium

The routine use of calcium during resuscitation is no longer recommended, as it may have detrimental effects in the ischaemic myocardium and may impair cerebral recovery (Resuscitation Council, UK, 2000). However, there are some situations when it should be considered. It is the treatment of choice to reverse respiratory depression or arrest due to magnesium toxicity during the treatment of pre-eclampsia/eclampsia (Doan-Wiggins, 1996), and it is also indicated in hypocalcaemia, hyperkalaemia and calcium channel blocker toxicity.

The dose is 10 ml of 10% calcium chloride i.v. Careful administration is required, as extravasion around the cannula may cause severe tissue injury. In addition, it will form an insoluble precipitate if mixed with sodium bicarbonate. It should not be administered via the tracheal route.

Sodium bicarbonate

Following a cardiac arrest, anaerobic cellular metabolism and the cessation of pulmonary gas exchange will lead to metabolic and respiratory acidosis respectively. In the past, sodium bicarbonate has been routinely used in resuscitation to 'correct' acidosis. However, there are numerous unwanted side effects of its administration; in pregnancy these include parodoxic fetal hypercarbia and acidosis (Doan-Wiggins, 1996). The optimum treatment for acidosis is effective ventilation and chest compressions, which in previously healthy individuals is normally quite sufficient to prevent a rapid or severe development of acidosis (Steedman and Robertson, 1992).

However, although the routine use of sodium bicarbonate is now discouraged (ERC, 1998), there are nevertheless situations when its use may be considered – for example, severe metabolic acidosis, cardiac arrest associated with hyperkalaemia, and tricyclic overdose (Resuscitation Council, UK, 2000).

The recommended dose is 50 mmol i.v. (50 ml of 8.4% solution). A flush with 0.9% sodium chloride should always precede and follow administration (sodium bicarbonate may inactivate other drugs). Careful administration is required, as extravasion around the cannula may cause severe tissue injury. Sodium bicarbonate cannot be administered via the tracheal route.

Emergency Caesarean section

Perimortem Caesarean section is one of the oldest known surgical procedures and dates back to the Roman era, when it was decreed in 715 BC that no woman in the latter stages of pregnancy could be buried without removing the baby first (Lattuada, 1952). Its incidence is actually quite rare, with only 300 reported cases since the late nineteenth century (Strong and Lowe, 1989).

During resuscitation, Caesarean section is not only an effort to save the life of the baby, but can also play an important role in the successful resuscitation of the mother (Morris and Willis, 1999). If there is potential fetal viability, perimortem Caesarean section should be performed promptly if initial attempts at resuscitation (including displacement of the gravid uterus) have failed to restore a circulation.

The timing is crucial, because the chances of infant survival decrease and the likelihood of neurological damage increase as the time interval from maternal arrest to Caesarean delivery rises. Although there is evidence that the fetus can tolerate prolonged periods of hypoxia (Windle, 1968), fetal survival and neurological outcome are optimum if Caesarean section is performed within 5 minutes of maternal arrest (Katz *et al.*, 1986). Although there have been reported cases of intact fetal survival following more than 20 minutes of maternal arrest (Katz *et al.*, 1986; Lopez-Zeno *et al.*, 1990), current recommendations advocate perimortem Caesarean section, if resuscitation is unsuccessful, within 5 minutes (Morris and Willis, 1994; Resuscitation Council, UK, 2000). For speed, a vertical abdominal and uterine incision should be used (Cox and Grady, 1999). Resuscitation should continue throughout the procedure (open cardiac massage should be considered).

It must be stressed that emergency Caesarean section may also improve the prognosis for the mother; maternal oxygen consumption will be reduced, venous return will improve, ventilation will be easier and resuscitation can be performed in the supine position (Cox and Grady, 1999).

Priorities of post-resuscitation care

The return of spontaneous circulation marks the beginning and not the end of a successful resuscitation. The end goal is a mother who has a normal cerebral function and a stable cardiac output and rhythm, together with adequate organ perfusion. In addition it is hoped that the fetus/baby will survive. If not already present, an obstetrician, anaesthetist, senior midwife and a paediatrician, if appropriate, should be called.

The priorities of post-resuscitation care include:

- rapid assessment of the mother's vital signs – airway, breathing and circulation – and support as appropriate
- determining the cause of the arrest – administer any necessary treatment to prevent a recurrence
- limiting organ damage – mean arterial blood pressure should be maintained at the mother's normal level, using appropriate inotropes and fluids if necessary
- monitoring the fetus/caring for the baby as appropriate
- undertaking any specific care (e.g. post-emergency Caesarean section management)
- transporting the mother to appropriate definitive care (normally an Intensive Care Unit)
- supporting members of the resuscitation team and the relatives.

Summary

This chapter has provided an overview of ALS in maternal resuscitation following Resuscitation Council (UK) guidelines. Specific interventions such as ECG monitoring, defibrillation, tracheal intubation, drugs and drug delivery have also been outlined. The possible need for prompt Caesarean section has been discussed.

Chapter 7

Anaphylaxis

Introduction

Anaphylaxis is an acute severe hypersensitivity reaction that can lead to asphyxia and cardiac arrest (Jevon, 2000). The incidence in pregnancy is not known. However, in the general population anaphylaxis seems to be on the increase, probably coinciding with a notable increase in the prevalence of allergic diseases in the last 30 years. It is often poorly managed; in particular, adrenaline is greatly under-used.

This had led to the publication of broad consensus guidelines by a Project Team of the Resuscitation Council (UK) (2000) on the appropriate emergency management of acute anaphylactic reactions by first medical responders. It must be stressed that these guidelines are not intended to replace existing advice for specific situations such as specialist clinics (Department of Health, 1996). Every midwife should be able to recognize the clinical features of anaphylaxis and be familiar with the initial emergency management.

The aim of this chapter is to provide an overview of the emergency medical treatment of anaphylactic reactions.

Objectives

By the end of the chapter the reader will be able to:

- define anaphylaxis
- discuss the pathophysiology of anaphylaxis
- list the causes of anaphylaxis
- describe the clinical features of anaphylaxis and discuss how to diagnose it
- discuss the management of anaphylaxis.

Definition

Anaphylaxis is an exaggerated response of a previously sensitized individual to a drug or substance, typically mediated by immunoglobulin (IgE). Anaphylactoid reactions are similar, but do not involve hypersensitivity. For this chapter the term anaphylaxis will be used to describe both types of reactions because the initial treatment will be the same; only the follow-up care will differ.

Pathogenesis

When exposed to a specific antigen, antigen-specific immunoglobulin E (IgE) antibodies, histamine and other vasoactive mediators are released from mast cells and basophils, producing circulatory, respiratory, gastrointestinal and cutaneous effects. These effects can include the development of pharyngeal and laryngeal oedema, bronchospasm, and decreased vascular tone and capillary leak causing circulatory collapse.

Causes of anaphylaxis

Causes include:

- insect stings
- certain foods – peanut and tree nuts are particularly dangerous (Ewan, 1996)
- blood products
- drugs – e.g. antibiotics, anaesthetic drugs
- immunizations
- contrast media
- latex protein allergy.

If the mother has a known latex protein allergy, products that contain latex should be identified and alternatives substituted. Products to be avoided include latex-containing gloves, Foley's indwelling catheters, blood infusion sets with a rubber injection site, Luer lock caps, rubber face masks, Entonox rubber tubing, elastic straps (e.g. those used with CTG monitoring), elastoplast, rubber coverings (e.g. for beds), sphygmomanometer tubing, and multidose bottles with rubber stoppers (Cox and Grady, 1999).

Clinical features and diagnosis

The lack of a consistent clinical picture can sometimes make an accurate diagnosis difficult. Anaphylactic reactions can vary in severity and the process can be slow, rapid or biphasic; occasionally the onset may be delayed by a few hours, and even persist for longer than 24 hours (Fisher, 1986). A detailed history and examination is essential as soon as possible. The clinical presentation often includes:

- urticarial rash
- tachycardia and hypotension
- pallor
- a sense of impending doom
- wheeze.

It is possible to mistake anaphylaxis for a panic attack or a vasovagal attack. A panic attack can lead to hyperventilation and, although there may be no hypotension, pallor, wheeze, or urticarial rash, an anxiety-related erythematous rash and tachycardia may be present. In a vasovagal attack, the absence of a rash, tachycardia and dyspnoea should rule out anaphylaxis as the cause of the collapse.

To prove that there is anaphylactic sensitivity to an allergen, a blood sample should be sent for estimation of serum trypase concentrations; an elevated serum trypase is seen following anaphylaxis. Ten millilitres of clotted blood should be taken, preferably 45–60 minutes following the reaction (up to 6 hours following the event is acceptable).

Management of anaphylaxis

Once anaphylaxis is suspected, senior medical help should be summoned and the mother reclined into a position of comfort (the supine position may help hypotension but exacerbate breathing difficulties). In late pregnancy, left lateral tilt should be used instead of the supine position. The flowchart (Figure 7.1) summarizes the current recommendations for the management of anaphylaxis (Project team of the Resuscitation Council UK, 2000).

Oxygen

If available, oxygen should be administered at a rate of 10–15 l/min, preferably via a face mask with an oxygen reservoir bag. This will allow delivery of approximately 90 per cent oxygen.

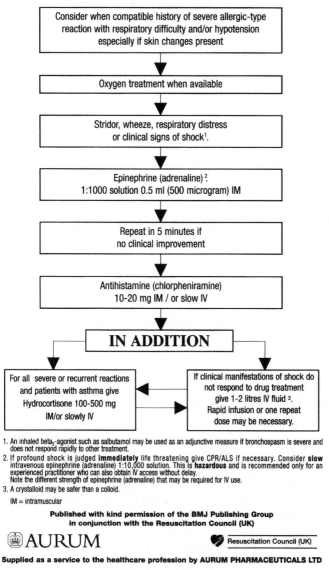

Anaphylactic Reactions for Adults
Treatment by First Medical Responders

Consider when compatible history of severe allergic-type reaction with respiratory difficulty and/or hypotension especially if skin changes present

▼

Oxygen treatment when available

▼

Stridor, wheeze, respiratory distress or clinical signs of shock[1].

▼

Epinephrine (adrenaline)[2]
1:1000 solution 0.5 ml (500 microgram) IM

▼

Repeat in 5 minutes if no clinical improvement

▼

Antihistamine (chlorpheniramine)
10-20 mg IM / or slow IV

▼

IN ADDITION

For all severe or recurrent reactions and patients with asthma give Hydrocortisone 100-500 mg IM/or slowly IV

If clinical manifestations of shock do not respond to drug treatment give 1-2 litres IV fluid [3].
Rapid infusion or one repeat dose may be necessary.

1. An inhaled beta₂-agonist such as salbutamol may be used as an adjunctive measure if bronchospasm is severe and does not respond rapidly to other treatment.
2. If profound shock is judged **immediately** life threatening give CPR/ALS if necessary. Consider **slow** intravenous epinephrine (adrenaline) 1:10,000 solution. This is **hazardous** and is recommended only for an experienced practitioner who can also obtain IV access without delay.
Note the different strength of epinephrine (adrenaline) that may be required for IV use.
3. A crystalloid may be safer than a colloid.

IM = intramuscular

Published with kind permission of the BMJ Publishing Group in conjunction with the Resuscitation Council (UK)

AURUM   Resuscitation Council (UK)

Supplied as a service to the healthcare profession by AURUM PHARMACEUTICALS LTD

Journal of Accident and Emergency Medicine 1999; 16(4)243-247
A report on the Emergency Medical Treatment of Anaphylactic Reactions
by a Project Team of the Resuscitation Council (UK)

Figure 7.1 Emergency management of anaphylaxis (reproduced with kind permission from the BMJ Publishing Group)

Epinephrine (adrenaline)

Epinephrine (adrenaline) is the most important drug in any severe anaphylactic reaction (Fisher, 1995). To be most effective, it should be given promptly (Patel *et al.*, 1994). It reverses peripheral vasodilation and reduces oedema (alpha receptor activity), dilates the airways, increases myocardial contractility, and suppresses histamine and leukotriene release.

The recommended dose is 500 µg i.m. (0.5 ml of 1 : 1000 solution). This can be repeated after 5 minutes if there is no improvement or if deterioration has occurred, particularly if the mother's consciousness level becomes or remains impaired in the presence of hypotension. Several doses may be required (*British National Formulary*, British Medical Association and Royal Pharmaceutical Society of Great Britain, 1999).

The intramuscular route is generally used for the administration of epinephrine, as it is relatively safe and adverse effects are rare. The more hazardous intravenous route is occasionally used, particularly if the patient is in profound shock which is immediately life threatening or in certain situations (e.g. anaesthesia). The 1 : 10 000 solution of adrenaline should be used in order to minimize complications, and the ECG closely monitored.

Self-administration of epinephrine

Individuals who are at considerable risk of anaphylaxis should carry adrenaline around with them at all times and be taught how to inject it. Two self-administration products are currently available; EpiPen® (Figure 7.2) and Anapen®. Both are fully assembled syringes that can deliver 300 µg of adrenaline i.m. Paediatric versions are also available; EpiPen Jr and Anapen Junior.

Cautions

1. To avoid a potentially dangerous interaction, the dose of adrenaline should be reduced in mothers who are taking tricyclic antidepressants or MAOIs (monoamine oxidase inhibitors).
2. The possibility of misinterpreting a panic or vasovagal attack for an anaphylaxis should be considered.
3. Two strengths of adrenaline are available; 1 : 1000 solution is used for i.m. injection, while the 1 : 10 000 solution is used for i.v. injection.
4. The subcutaneous route for the administration of adrenaline should not be utilized, because absorption is considerably slower (Simons *et al.*, 1998).

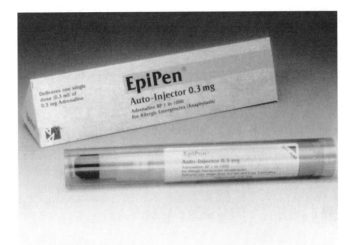

Figure 7.2 Epipen®

Antihistamines

An antihistamine such as chlorpheniramine (Piriton) should be used routinely in all anaphylactic reactions, although care should be taken to avoid drug-induced hypotension. The recommended dose is 10–20 mg, either i.m. or by slow i.v. injection.

Hydrocortisone

Hydrocortisone should be administered following severe anaphylactic reactions to help prevent late sequelae, particularly in asthmatics who have been on corticosteroidal treatment previously. The recommended dose is 100–500 mg, either i.m. or by slow i.v. injection. Again, care should be taken to avoid inducing further hypotension.

Fluids

If severe hypotension fails to respond rapidly to drug therapy, fluids should be infused. A crystalloid may be safer than a colloid (Schierhout and Roberts, 1998), and a rapid infusion of 1–2 litres may be required.

Follow-up

Even if the reaction is only moderate, the mother should be warned of the possibility of an early recurrence of symptoms. Sometimes the mother will need to be monitored for 8–24 hours, particularly when the reaction:

- is severe and is of slow onset due to idiopathic anaphylaxis
- occurs in a severe asthmatic
- is complicated by a severe asthmatic attack
- could again be triggered because further absorption of the allergen is possible.

Summary

Anaphylaxis can be life threatening. This chapter has detailed the broad consensus guidelines by a Project Team of the Resuscitation Council (UK) (1999) on the appropriate emergency management of acute anaphylactic reactions by first medical responders. Every midwife should be able to recognize the clinical features of anaphylaxis and be familiar with the initial emergency management.

Chapter 8

Records and record keeping

Introduction

An accurate written record detailing the resuscitation event is essential. It forms an integral part of the medical and midwifery management of the mother, and can help to protect the practitioner if defence of his or her actions is required. Unfortunately, the exact timing and sequence of events and interventions can sometimes be difficult to recall. Despite this, accurate record keeping will still be expected.

The aim of this chapter is to discuss some of the principles of good record keeping, with particular reference to maternal resuscitation.

Objectives

By the end of the chapter the reader will be able to:

- discuss the importance of accurate record keeping
- outline the principles of effective record keeping
- detail what should be included in post-resuscitation records
- discuss when the records become a legal document
- discuss the procedure for the reporting of proven or suspected amniotic fluid embolism.

Importance of accurate record keeping

Accurate record keeping will help to protect the welfare of the mother by promoting high standards of clinical care and continuity of care through better communication and dissemination of information between members of the inter-professional health care team. Accurate records will also help the practitioner to promptly detect any changes in the mother's condition.

Principles of effective record keeping

According to the UKCC (1998a; Figure 8.1), there are a number of factors which contribute to effective record keeping. The records should:

- be factual, consistent and accurate
- be documented as soon as possible after the event, providing current information on the care and condition of the mother and fetus/baby
- be documented clearly and in such a way that the text cannot be erased
- have any alterations and additions dated, timed and signed, with all original entries clearly legible
- be accurately dated, timed and signed (including a printed signature)
- not include abbreviations, jargon, meaningless phrases or irrelevant speculation.

Resuscitation records – what to include

It is most important that the resuscitation attempt is fully documented in the notes. The following should be included:

- time of arrest, including presenting ECG rhythm
- details of resuscitation, including ECG rhythms and response to treatment
- tracheal intubation time and duration of ventilation
- details of drugs administered, including doses and routes used
- details of defibrillation
- any pertinent blood chemistry, e.g. arterial blood gases, pH and base deficit results
- names of personnel present, including designation
- reasons for any delay in resuscitation
- details of communication with the relatives
- when resuscitation was stopped, either because it was successful or because it was abandoned
- relevant fetal/baby details.

The clinical records should be legible, and accurately reflect what happened during the resuscitation attempt. A standardized form for recording resuscitation events may help ensure that a complete record is made.

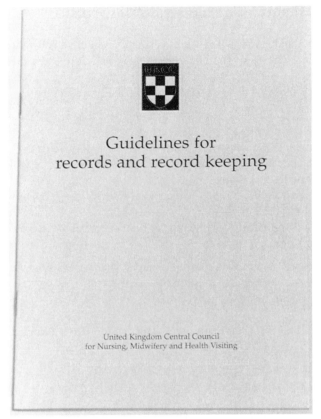

Figure 8.1   *Guidelines for Records and Record Keeping* (UKCC 1998)

Records as a legal document

There is often concern as to what constitutes a legal document. Basically, any document requested by the court becomes a legal document (Dimond, 1994); midwifery records, medical records, X-rays, laboratory reports – in fact, any document that may be relevant to the case. If any of the documents are missing, the writer of the records may be cross-examined as to the circumstances of their disappearance (Dimond, 1994):

> Medical records are not proof of the truth of the facts stated in them but the maker of the records may be called to give evidence as to the truth as to what is contained in them.

The UK amniotic fluid embolism register

A confidential register of all cases of amniotic fluid embolism in the UK has been established. The aim is to identify any differences or common factors associated with survival and fatality, which may then perhaps help to reduce the number of maternal deaths from this condition.

The entry criteria are:

- acute hypertension or cardiac arrest
- acute hypoxia (dyspnoea, cyanosis or respiratory arrest)
- coagulopathy (laboratory evidence of intravascular coagulation or severe haemorrhage)
- onset of all the above during labour or Caesarean section, or within 30 minutes of delivery
- no other clinical condition or potential explanation for the signs and symptoms.

All cases of suspected or proven amniotic fluid embolism, whether the mother has survived or not, should be reported to:

Mr Derek Tuffnell
Consultant Obstetrician
Bradford Royal Infirmary
Duckworth Lane
Bradford BD9 6RJ
Tel. 01274 364520 Fax 01274 366690

Summary

The importance of accurate records following a maternal resuscitation attempt cannot be stressed enough. The records must be:

- factual
- legible
- clear
- concise
- accurate
- signed, timed and dated.

Chapter 9

Reporting and managing a maternal death

Introduction

The *Confidential Enquiries into Maternal Deaths* is a triennial report from the Department of Health which provides an overview of the numbers and causes of maternal deaths in the United Kingdom. The information and data, which are collated and anonymized, identify where improvements can be made in clinical practice or in the provision of the service, which may then help to prevent maternal deaths in the future. It is therefore important to ensure that every maternal death is notified promptly, following national guidelines, so that all the information on each case is readily available.

Professionals who are involved in providing maternal care, in both the primary and secondary care setting, must understand what constitutes a maternal death and the procedure that needs to be followed in the event of one. The aim of this chapter is to understand the procedure that needs to be followed when reporting and managing a maternal death based on West Midland's Regional Guidelines (Noble, 1997).

Objectives

By the end of the chapter the reader will be able to:

- discuss the aims of the *Confidential Enquiries into Maternal Deaths*
- define what constitutes a maternal death
- discuss a suggested procedure for the management of maternal death in the hospital environment
- outline the notification procedure following a maternal death

- discuss the suggested procedure for the management of a maternal death in the primary care setting
- briefly outline the procedure for completion of the Enquiry form.

Aims of the *Confidential Enquiries into Maternal Deaths*

The aims of the enquiries are to:

- assess the main causes of, and trends in, maternal deaths; to identify any avoidable or substandard factors; to promulgate these findings to all relevant health care professionals
- reduce maternal mortality and morbidity rates, as well as the proportion of cases due to substandard care
- make recommendations concerning the improvement of clinical care and service provision, including local audit, to purchasers of obstetric services and professionals involved in caring for pregnant women
- suggest directions for future areas for research and audit at local and national level
- produce a triennial report for the four Chief Medical Officers of the United Kingdom.

Definitions of maternal death

A maternal death is any death that occurs during or within 1 year of pregnancy, childbirth or abortion and which is directly or indirectly related to these conditions.

A *direct maternal death* is a death that results from obstetric complications of the pregnant state (pregnancy, labour and puerperium), for example from interventions, omissions, incorrect treatment or from a chain of events resulting from any of the these.

An *indirect maternal death* is a death that results from a previous existing disease, or from a disease which developed during pregnancy and was not due to direct obstetric causes but was aggravated by the physiological effects of pregnancy.

A *fortuitous death* is a death that results from unrelated causes that just happen to occur during pregnancy or puerperium (e.g. a road traffic accident).

A *late death* is one that occurs between 42 days and 1 year following an abortion, miscarriage or delivery and is due to direct or indirect maternal causes.

Management of an in-hospital maternal death

The Trust Chief Executive should be informed and one person should be appointed who has overall responsibility to ensure that the local policies are followed. A co-ordinator should also be nominated, usually a senior midwife, a supervisor of midwives or a consultant obstetrician.

Role of the co-ordinator

The role of the co-ordinator can be complex and demanding. He or she must ensure that a confidential, accurate record of each section of the procedure is followed and, if necessary, must be released from his/her normal duties. A checklist should be drawn up to ensure that the following is actioned:

- nomination of an experienced member of staff to support the woman's family; this person will also be the main point of contact for the relatives to prevent conflicting information being passed on
- notification of the on-call consultant, who should be asked to see the woman's relatives as soon as possible (if the woman already has a named consultant, he or she should also be informed)
- notification of supervisor of midwives (UKCC, 1998b), if not already nominated to be the co-ordinator.

Post-mortem

The Mortuary Department and the on-call pathologist should be notified. Guidelines for maternal autopsy are available from the Royal College of Pathologists. If at all possible, a post-mortem should be undertaken to confirm the cause of death; the consultant should seek permission for this from the mother's next-of-kin. The coroner will need to be informed if the cause of death is unknown; he or she will then be responsible for requesting a post-mortem.

Case notes and documentation

All the case notes should be completed, photocopied and secured as soon as possible. If there is a hearing on the case, the coroner will request the case notes and all the documentation. Where appropriate, the local Untoward Incident Policy should be followed and an internal audit into the events surrounding the death carried out.

Staff support

Staff involved in the case may also require support, for example from the chaplain or staff counsellor. This should be provided if necessary.

Registering the dead baby

In the event of the baby dying *in utero*, the following need to be taken into account:

1. The removal of a dead baby from its dead mother during the post-mortem is not classified as a stillbirth, because the post-mortem is being carried out on the mother rather than the baby. In these circumstances, it is not a legal requirement to register the baby. However, the expressed wishes of the next-of-kin need to be taken into account. The medical practitioner may therefore issue a death certificate to enable the family to register the baby as stillborn. The majority of Registrars of Births, Marriages and Deaths will comply, but local policies regarding this issue need to be agreed in order to avoid confusion and further distress to the family.

2. As most pathologists will remove the baby at post-mortem, it would be sensible to follow the local stillbirth/neonatal procedure whether the baby is to be registered as a death or not. In addition, the normal procedure for reporting infant deaths to the Confidential Enquiry (CESDI) should be followed.

Religious considerations

If requested, the local priest, vicar, rabbi or appropriate other should be contacted. If the family is uncertain or would just like someone of faith to be with them, the hospital chaplain should be notified.

Other practitioners who need to be notified

The following should also be notified:

- clinical managers within the department, when next on duty, particularly as they may later be involved with the case
- The general practitioner and the community midwives involved in the mother's care.

Meeting the consultant

Arrangements should be made for the family to see the consultant at the earliest opportunity. At least one further meeting should be arranged once all the results from the investigations, post-mortem etc. are available so that the findings can be comprehensively discussed and explained.

Notification procedure following a maternal death

The following should be notified of the death:

- the coroner, if the cause of death is unknown
- the 'coroner's officer', who may insist on being present when the family view the body (bodies) in the mortuary; if this situation arises, sensitive handling and organization will be required
- the Director of Public Health of the Health Authority in which the maternal death has occurred; the responsibility for notification rests with the consultant, midwife or general practitioner who had overall responsibility for the pregnancy, or the consultant or general practitioner treating the woman during her final illness if the death occurred within 1 year following the end of her pregnancy
- the CESDI co-ordinator at the Regional Perinatal Audit Office if the death of a baby has occurred
- the mother's general practitioner and health visitor
- the Local Supervising Authority Officer
- if the woman had been admitted having been treated or booked in another area, the senior midwife and consultant in that hospital
- if the woman was not resident in the hospital's local district, the local Director of Public Health should notify his or her counterpart in the area of the woman's residence
- if the death has occurred outside the Maternity Unit, the consultant, general practitioner or midwife in charge of the pregnancy should be informed
- Social Services if the family social circumstances are applicable, or if a live baby needs support
- the Registrar of Births and Deaths – if possible, the attending doctor must promptly and accurately complete a death certificate and give it to the relatives to pass on.

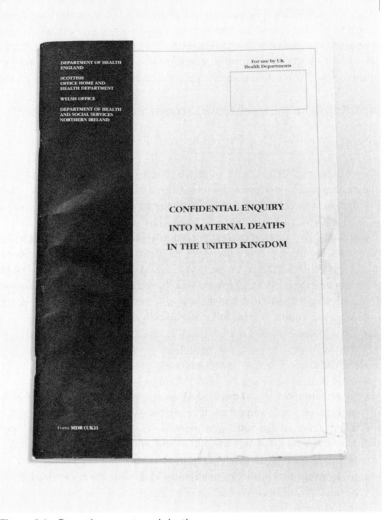

Figure 9.1 Reporting a maternal death

Managing a maternal death in primary care

The general practitioner should notify the Director of Public Health and the consultant obstetrician if the mother had delivered or had received care at the hospital. Guidance should be available in each general practice to ensure that all the staff in the primary care team have access to and understand the procedure to be followed in the event of a maternal death. This guidance should reflect the recommendations outlined above on the definition of a maternal death and responsibility for reporting a maternal death.

Completion of the Confidential Enquiry form

On being notified of a maternal death, the local Director of Public Health should request a Confidential Enquiry Form (Figure 9.1) from the CEMD Principal Medical Officer at the Department of Health (tel. 020 7972 4344), and have as many details as possible at hand.

Once the initial details of the case have been completed, the form should be passed to the clinicians involved for local completion (it would be helpful if one person co-ordinated this). After completion the form should be returned to the Director of Public Health, who will then forward it to the Regional Assessor. In order to preserve anonymity, no photocopies of the Confidential Enquiry form should be made at any time.

Summary

It is essential to identify and establish the facts surrounding maternal deaths accurately. It is most important that all the Confidential Enquiries are undertaken according to national standards and expectations, and this may then help to reduce the incidence of maternal deaths. This chapter has provided an outline of how these enquiries should be carried out, based on current guidance from the West Midlands NHS Executive (Noble, 1997).

Chapter 10

Bereavement

Introduction

Sudden death, which is recognized as one of the most traumatic events that can be experienced, can leave bereaved relatives struggling to cope with their feelings and reactions (Wright, 1996). Supporting bereaved relatives is never easy, especially in the tragic event of a maternal death (Mander, 1994). Nevertheless, health care professionals need to know how to help people through the process of grieving. Early correct handling of those who have been suddenly bereaved can greatly ease their journey through the phases of grief and help reduce complications (Resuscitation Council, UK, 2000).

The aim of this chapter is to provide an introduction to the general principles of managing bereavement. A more comprehensive and detailed account can be found elsewhere (Wright, 1996).

Objectives

By the end of this chapter the reader will be able to:

- describe an ideal layout for the relatives' room
- discuss how to break bad news
- discuss the principles of telephone notification of relatives
- discuss the issues involved with relatives witnessing resuscitation.

Relatives' room

The relatives' room should be spacious, well lit and, if possible, have a window to the outside. This will help to reduce relatives' feelings of claustrophobia and isolation (Bury Medical Audit, 1994). In addition, it is recommended (British Association of A & E Medicine and the Royal College of Nursing, 1994) that the relatives' room should have the following:

- comfortable domestic chairs and sofas, including provision for people with special needs
- ashtrays (if smoking is permitted)
- a telephone with direct dial-in and dial-out facilities and telephone directories
- a wash basin with soap, towel, mirror, freshen-up pack and tissues
- a television/radio available but not prominent
- hot and cold drinks, a refrigerator, kettle and a non-institutional tea/ coffee set
- books and toys for children
- access to toilet facilities.

Breaking bad news
Who should tell the relatives?

If the relatives are not present when the mother dies, or if they arrive after her death, somebody will have to break the news to them. Certainly when the death is unexpected the most senior doctor available, with a senior midwife in support, should tell the relatives. The doctor is then at hand to answer the inevitable questions concerning the mode of death and what was done to try and prevent it. In some situations when the death is expected, the senior midwife may be the best person to tell the relatives.

Preparation

Adequate preparation is essential. All the relevant information regarding the deceased, including medical and resuscitation details, should be gathered together. Self-preparation, e.g. washing hands, checking clothing for blood, is also important. The name of the closest relative of the deceased should be determined.

Communication with the relatives

- Introduce yourself and colleague(s), confirm that they are the correct relatives and identify who is the closest relative.

- Sit down in order to be at the same level as the relatives; establish and maintain eye contact.
- Allow time, do not rush, and allow periods of silence so that the information can be absorbed.
- Avoid platitudes such as 'I know what you are going through'; rather, reflect back on their emotions – for example, 'it must be a terrible shock for you'.
- Answer questions in a sympathetic and non-judgmental way.

What to tell the relatives

The way bad news is broken is critical. Words like 'dead' or 'died' are unequivocal and will not be misinterpreted. Honest direct information about the sequence of events, from practitioners who do not skirt around the real issues, is valued by relatives (Wright, 1996).

The use of euphemisms is not recommended. The following phrases, although well meaning, may lead to misinterpretation:

- 'she has passed on'
- 'she has slipped away'
- 'she has gone to a better place' (to another hospital?)
- 'we have lost her'.

Telephone notification of relatives

Notifying the relatives by telephone can be difficult. To minimize confusion and misunderstanding, the information should be clear and concise. The following is recommended:

- Identify yourself and the hospital.
- Establish who you are speaking to – if this is not the key relative, find out where he or she can be found.
- Give the name of the patient and her condition. It seems to be common practice not to inform relatives over the telephone that the patient has died, but instead to tell them that the patient's condition has deteriorated rapidly or is critical, or words to that effect. A dilemma arises if the relatives ask over the telephone whether their loved one has died. The authors' view is that an honest approach is preferable. Wright (1996) suggests that if the hospital is easily accessible, tell the relatives when they arrive and not over the phone.

- Check that the relatives are clear about the message and that they are familiar with how to get to the hospital.
- Document the exact details of the telephone conversation.

Relatives present during resuscitation

Being separated from a loved one, particularly at the time of death, can cause considerable distress (Renner, 1991). Should relatives therefore be present during resuscitation? This subject has been extensively debated in the literature in recent years. Some doctors believe that relatives should be allowed to witness the resuscitation attempt (Adams *et al.*, 1994). Others point out that having relatives present can cause anxiety for junior doctors, other staff and also for the relatives themselves, particularly if invasive procedures are being undertaken (Schilling, 1994; Zoltie *et al.*, 1994).

The Resuscitation Council UK advise that, although the feelings of staff must be considered, the prime consideration should be for the relatives and their expressed wishes. If relatives are present during resuscitation, a designated member of staff should accompany them and explain the procedures (Chalk, 1995).

Summary

Health care professionals need to know how to support bereaved relatives through the process of grieving following a maternal death. This chapter discussed the principles of the early management of bereavement, including how to break bad news.

Chapter 11

Ethical and legal issues

Introduction

When resuscitation is required, it must be instigated promptly following national recommendations (European Resuscitation Council, 1998). It is also important to recognize when such measures should be withheld. Consequently, there are a number of ethical and legal issues faced by practitioners who may be involved in maternal resuscitation. In the current NHS climate, with increasing risks of litigation, it is important for practitioners to ensure that they are able to justify their actions and provide a reasonable standard of care.

The aim of this chapter is to discuss some of the ethical and legal issues in maternal resuscitation faced by medical and midwifery staff. It must be emphasized that only a brief insight into these issues can be provided in such a short chapter, and further reading is essential if a comprehensive understanding is required or if policies and procedures need to be formulated (Dimond, 1994).

Objectives

By the end of this chapter the reader will be able to:

- discuss what is meant by a 'reasonable standard of care'
- discuss the criteria for making 'do not resuscitate' orders
- describe measures to manage the legal risks associated with maternal resuscitation.

Standard of care

A practitioner (e.g. a midwife or obstetrician) owes a 'duty of care' to a mother in need of resuscitation, and is expected to provided a reasonable standard of care. Although at present there is no English precedent, it is quite possible, as has happened in the USA, that in the future patients and relatives may win claims for compensation for injury sustained during a resuscitation attempt if clinical negligence can be proved.

The key issue considered by courts regarding clinical negligence litigation claims is the expectation that the patient should have received a reasonable standard of care. Such standards will become increasingly higher in line with the objectives of the Government and clinical governance. When determining whether this standard of care has been breached during any aspect of the resuscitation process, the level of experience and expertise that the practitioner has or is expected to have, together with the circumstances, will be taken into account (Resuscitation Council, UK, 2000):

> A claim of inexperience or lack of training will not be successful as a defence in an allegation of negligence if a practitioner has been called upon only to work within the limits of his own expected competence.

On the other hand, if:

> an inexperienced practitioner is obliged to commence emergency treatment, but at the same time calls for specialist help, his lack of training will normally be a defence if his performance is suboptimal.

In the above circumstances, the practitioner should consider the availability of more skilled help and should exercise a cautious degree of intervention within the realms of his or her own skills and training. It is also important to mention that where an expert practitioner takes control of a resuscitation procedure and delegates tasks to more junior members of staff within that team, that practitioner will remain accountable for any suboptimal treatment delivered by the junior member of staff if the same was outside their range of experience and training, although where there is a reckless or negligent acceptance of a delegated task there is a liability on the practitioner accepting the task when the result is harm to the patient.

In order to ascertain whether there has been a breach of duty, demonstrated by a fall in the standard of care delivered, it is first of all necessary to establish exactly what standard should have been followed, and whether the defendant's actions differed (if at all) from what it was reasonable to expect (Dimond, 1994), to the detriment of the patient. The Resuscitation Council UK have set a standard of care with the publication of basic and advanced life support guidelines (Resuscitation Council, UK, 2000). The courts are likely to expect medical and midwifery staff to ensure that they perform resuscitation to this standard – within, of course, their capabilities and experience:

It is important that practitioners should not take on responsibility beyond the level to which they have been trained.

To determine the legal standard expected from practitioners, the courts apply the so-called Bolam test, which derives from a case decided in 1957. It was in the Bolam case (Bolam *v* Friern Barnet, HMC 1957, 2 All ER 118) that the standard was first described as:

'when there is a situation which involves the use of some special skill or competence, then the test as to whether there has been negligence or not is . . . the standard of the ordinary skilled man exercising and professing to have that special skill. A man need not possess the highest expert skill; it is well established that it is sufficient if he exercises the ordinary skill of an ordinary competent man exercising that particular art.'

It was also stated in the Bolam case that:

a doctor is not negligent if he is acting in accordance with a practice accepted as proper by a reasonable body of medical men skilled in that art

and further he is not necessarily negligent

merely because there is a body of such opinion that takes a contrary view.

(The Bolam test, of course, applies to all health care professionals, not just medical staff.)

Therefore, the approach a practitioner decides to adopt during maternal resuscitation may not necessarily be negligent in all circumstances. However, deviating from nationally recognized guidelines would require clear explanation and justification as to why the guidelines did not apply in those particular circumstances, should the patient suffer harm as a result.

When considering guidelines and protocols for resuscitation, the practitioner must always bear in mind the best interests of the patient. If applying a standard method of treatment supported by a protocol or guideline is clearly not relevant to the patient's needs but the practitioner blindly follows the protocol, resulting in an adverse outcome for the patient, then the practitioner would be culpable under the Bolam principle. In the Airedale Hospitals NHS Trust *v* Bland case (1994), the court found that the medical staff who had followed the withdrawal of treatment guidelines published by the GMC were not negligent because the guidelines satisfied the Bolam test. The judges took pains to point out that, had the guidelines not been in line with current accepted practice, the blind following of them would not have protected the Trust against a finding of negligence.

In the more recent case of Bolitho *v* City and Hackney Hospital (1998), the court considered the sensibility of the application of the Bolam test for the first time since 1957. The judges held that it could not simply be the case that where there was support for defendant doctors' actions through a responsible body of medical opinion, that doctor would not be negligent. The supporting opinion itself must be capable of logical analysis and commonsensical application.

For the Bolam test, this means that there is an additional criterion to a doctor not being negligent merely because there is a body of opinion with a contrary view. Whilst this is still true, the converse is that a doctor may still be negligent even if there is a body of medical opinion which takes a supportive view, unless that body of opinion can convince the court that it is reasonable in all the circumstances. According to Dimond (1994), there are a number of lessons to be learnt from court cases in relation to expected standards of care. In particular, the practitioner must be familiar with current standards of practice. This includes being aware of protocols, guidelines and procedures that have been drawn up locally and nationally, and keeping abreast of changes and updates.

Despite the availability of guidelines, there is still room for professional judgement and discretion. However, clear and precise records need to be kept detailing the particular circumstances and justifications for departing from approved protocols and standards.

The practitioner's knowledge and skills should be kept up to date because, under clinical governance and Government initiatives for the improvement of health care, standards of care are likely to rise. The practitioner will be judged against the standard most universally applied at the time of the incident. In this context, the practitioner should be aware that where there are conflicting standards the courts will often prefer the one which was most least likely to result in harm to the patient.

An appropriate standard of care is also expected from the professional bodies. In the Midwives Rules and Code of Practice (UKCC, 1998) it states that:

> you should be appropriately prepared and clinically up to date to ensure that you are able effectively to carry out emergency procedures for the mother or baby such as resuscitation.

In addition:

> each practitioner retains the clinical accountability for her own practice.

'Do not resuscitate' orders

Although resuscitation will nearly always be undertaken in the event of a maternal cardiac arrest, there will be occasions when a cardiac arrest represents a terminal event in a mother's illness and therefore resuscitation would probably be inappropriate (unless being undertaken while a Caesarean section was being performed to save a baby). It is therefore important to identify any mothers for whom resuscitation would be inappropriate and probably futile. Recent guidelines (BMA *et al.*, 1999) recommend that CPR should not be undertaken when:

- the patient's condition indicates that effective CPR is unlikely to be successful
- CPR is not in accordance with the recorded sustained wishes of a mentally competent patient
- successful CPR is unlikely to result in a length and quality of life acceptable to the patient.

The decision not to resuscitate should be raised and discussed if any of the above conditions apply. Although the senior clinician in charge of the mother's care (usually the consultant obstetrician) is ultimately responsible for making the decision, the opinions of midwives and other members of the team should also be sought. In addition, the mother and relatives should be consulted where appropriate.

When a "do not resuscitate" order is made, it must be clearly documented in the mother's medical notes by the most senior clinician present. It should be dated and signed, and should include the rationale behind the decision and when it should be reviewed. In addition, it should be documented in the nursing/midwifery notes. It is also important that the records accurately reflect the wishes of the mother, expressed when she is legally and mentally competent, or, when these circumstances do not apply, the views of the mother's next of kin or other significant persons (Dimond, 1994) – although the latter are not legally binding on the practitioner.

It would be prudent for the midwife to check that what has been actually documented in the medical and midwifery notes actually reflects any conversations regarding a "do not resuscitate" order, as discrepancies can and do occur. Accurate record keeping is essential, because it will protect the welfare of the mother by promoting better communication and dissemination of information between members of the health care team (UKCC, 1998). If the mother's prognosis or expressed wishes change and the "do not resuscitate" order is no longer appropriate, the midwife should bring this to the attention of medical colleagues as soon as possible so that the order can be reviewed.

Refusal of consent to be resuscitated

If the mother withdraws her consent to be resuscitated should the occasion arise, this should also be clearly documented in the medical notes and signed by both herself and an independent witness. This decision should be respected, but is only legally binding on the practitioner subject to the following caveats:

1. The practitioner's duty is always to act in the best interest of their patients.
2. In considering the validity of the refusal, the practitioner should have serious regard for the mental capacity of the patient at the time the refusal was made.
3. The practitioner should ensure that the patient has full understanding of the consequences of their refusal, and document clearly the details of any conversation.
4. If in doubt of the patient's understanding of the order, the practitioner should seek legal advice or, in an emergency, resuscitate. It is unlikely that in these circumstances the court would support penalizing a clinician for saving a life, unless the prognosis and circumstances were such that no other clinician would have resuscitated.

Advance directives

To date, the legal effectiveness of advance directives has not been put to the test in English Courts. The Resuscitation Council, UK (2000) has suggested that there is no reason to believe that the advance directive is invalid if:

- it was intended to apply in the circumstances arising
- the maker was mentally competent at the time it was made
- the maker was not under someone else's influence; and
- the maker was fully aware of the relevant risks.

However, in the absence of a full discussion between the patient and the clinician immediately prior to an arrest or terminal phase of the patient's health it is for the clinician to decide and assess whether the patient did in fact intend the advance directive to apply to a given set of circumstances. This is complicated by the fact that the patient may well have lost the capacity to revoke an earlier decision.

Risk management strategy

Professionals can take a risk management approach to litigation which on the one hand ensures high standards of care and on the other high standards of evidence should litigation be threatened.

Henderson and Jones (1996) have described the key components of a risk management strategy to minimize the risk of litigation:

- standards of care
- use of protocols
- monitoring practice
- identifying risk activities
- keeping records
- responding to complaints
- maintaining a safe environment.

These points will now be discussed in turn in the context of maternal resuscitation.

Standards of care

The law and the public will expect the practitioner to attain a recognized standard of care that would be expected from any competent health care professional. The practitioner will therefore need to keep up-to-date with current guidelines and strive to ensure that, whenever possible, practice is based on evidence. This will of course require not only knowledge, but also, and certainly more importantly, competency at resuscitation skills. Training and regular updates in resuscitation techniques are therefore essential if this required level of competency is to be not only reached but also maintained.

There should also be an audit system in place to ensure that these standards are being achieved and maintained. One possible and objective way of undertaking this is through scenario testing using a manikin, preferably in the clinical area, following recommended guidelines. It is certain to be more beneficial if the team approach to resuscitation is evaluated, and it is therefore desirable to encourage participation of the obstetrician, crash team and the midwife together. This will help provide a realistic situation.

Protocols

Protocols (e.g. who should attend a maternal arrest) can help to reduce the risk of error and ensure that the desired standard of care is delivered. Where appropriate, they should be based on current research, guidelines and recommendations, and should be determined and agreed locally. It is important that all practitioners who will be expected to follow them are involved in their production, as this will help to ensure that they are followed.

Monitoring practice

All resuscitation attempts should be audited. This can be done either by completing a standard audit form immediately following the event (the preferred method), or retrospectively by reviewing the mother's notes. The main purpose of the audit is to identify any problems (e.g. with equipment or with the resuscitation procedure) and rectify them accordingly. Potential problems may also be highlighted.

Identifying risk activities

Risk activities should be identified – for example, the decision as to when to request medical support during resuscitation is one area of clinical practice that is prone to or favours successful litigation. It is important to ensure that regular training is undertaken, and that appropriate protocols are not only in place but are also regularly reviewed.

Keeping records

The keeping of clear and comprehensive records is part of the duty of care owed to the mother (Dimond, 1994). In addition, these records are invaluable in providing evidence in cases of litigation. It is therefore imperative to ensure that high standards of record keeping are maintained. It is worth noting that there are national guidelines on record keeping – for example, *Guidelines for records and record keeping* (UKCC, 1998a).

Responding to complaints

Ideally, complaints should be investigated and settled at an early stage. This may prevent them from becoming formal complaints. Good communication and explanations may also reduce the incidence of complaints in the first place.

Maintaining a safe environment

The requirements of the Health and Safety at Work Act (1974) should, of course, be followed. Care must particularly be taken with sharps and body fluids. Regular checks should be carried out on the resuscitation equipment, following the manufacturers' recommendations, and any faults or defects reported and rectified.

Summary

If resuscitation is required, it is essential to undertake it promptly and effectively. However, it is just as important to recognize when these measures should be withheld. The practitioner must be aware of these ethical and legal dilemmas, and ensure that a reasonable standard of care in maternal resuscitation is provided.

Chapter 12

Resuscitation training

Introduction

Resuscitation employs skills that are essentially practical, and practitioners need hands-on training both to acquire and to maintain their skills. The methods used to teach resuscitation techniques have been the subject of much investigation in recent years. Teachers and educationalists have devoted considerable effort to determining the optimum method of teaching resuscitation techniques so that the necessary skills are both acquired and easily retained. In addition, resuscitation training has been enhanced by the availability of advanced and realistic training manikins and models.

The aim of this chapter is to outline how resuscitation training can best be provided.

Objectives

By the end of the chapter the reader will be able to:

- discuss why resuscitation training is important
- state national recommendations for resuscitation training
- state the key learning objectives of resuscitation training
- discuss how training can be provided
- discuss the evaluation of resuscitation training
- describe what training manikins and models are currently available for resuscitation training.

The importance of resuscitation training

Resuscitation training is important for three main reasons:

1. Practitioners' skills in resuscitation are often very poor (Lowenstein *et al.*, 1981; Wynne *et al.*, 1987)

2. Rather worryingly, there is considerable disparity between perceived competence and the actual ability to undertake effective resuscitation (Smith and Hatchett, 1992)
3. The experience of senior practitioners attending cardiac arrests is that confidence levels are often high, but this is generally not matched by high skill levels (Wynne *et al.*, 1987).

It has also been demonstrated that retention of resuscitation skills is very poor (McKenna and Glendon, 1985), and a significant deterioration in competence has been shown after only 10 weeks. At present there is unfortunately no consensus on the best way to overcome this problem, nor on how often refresher training is required. Certainly the more frequent the updates the better, though realistically an annual update is probably the most achievable.

National recommendations for resuscitation training

The Royal College of Physician's Report (1987) *Resuscitation from Cardiopulmonary Arrest: Training and Organization* recommended that all obstetric staff should be trained in basic resuscitation techniques. The *Confidential Enquiries into Maternal Deaths 1988–90* (Department of Health, 1993) emphasized that new medical and midwifery staff should have an induction course, and that their continuing education programme should include regular rehearsals of emergency procedures, especially in resuscitation. More recently, the *Confidential Enquiries into Maternal Deaths 1993–96* (Department of Health, 1998) recommended that 'all clinical staff, including consultants, should attend local resuscitation courses', and that 'units should consider the possibility of undertaking multidisciplinary practice sessions'.

It is therefore expected that all obstetric staff should receive training in maternal resuscitation. However, a recent study suggests that only 42 per cent of senior midwives and 33 per cent of junior midwives receive formal training (Department of Health, 1998). All Maternity Units should address this issue and ensure that staff are trained following national recommendations.

The key learning objectives

Suggested key learning objectives, which may help in the provision of a training session in maternal resuscitation, are listed below.

At the end of the training session the learner will be able to:

- demonstrate the correct procedure for checking emergency equipment
- demonstrate the correct procedure for assessing a collapsed, apparently lifeless mother
- state the correct procedure for summoning senior help
- demonstrate the correct procedure for opening and maintaining a clear airway
- demonstrate the correct procedure for insertion of an oropharyngeal airway
- demonstrate the correct procedure for bag/valve/mask resuscitation, and achieve chest rise on the manikin
- demonstrate how to relieve aortocaval compression
- demonstrate effective chest compressions on a manikin, achieving a rate of 100 per minute
- describe the correct procedure for cricoid pressure
- list the equipment required for intubation
- list four complications of intubation
- demonstrate how to attach the defibrillator and select lead 2
- specify the indications for administering adrenaline
- discuss when resuscitation should be stopped
- discuss the possible indications for withholding resuscitation measures
- discuss the process of constant reassessment during a resuscitation attempt.

Resuscitation training methods

Adults are usually well motivated to learn once they realize that the course content is relevant to them. In addition, adults generally learn best when they are treated as adults and when their skills, experience and prior knowledge are recognized and utilized.

Considerable research has been undertaken evaluating the principles of teaching basic and advanced resuscitation skills and factors affecting their retention. Both the course content and the time devoted to practice on manikins will influence skill attainment and subsequent retention of skills (Wynne *et al.*, 1999). In addition, constructive feedback during training is important and should not only identify the student's strong points, which will increase the students' confidence and motivation, but also identify any weaknesses or deficiencies that need to be addressed and require more practice. Ridicule of students in the event of poor performance should be avoided.

There are various methods of providing resuscitation training, and the methods chosen will be dependent upon a number of factors including time allocation, number of instructors, number of students, equipment, facilities and learning objectives. Some of these methods are described below.

Lectures

Lectures can be used to revise core material, highlight key points and complement practical stations, but should not replace practical teaching on manikins and models. They also provide a valuable opportunity for group discussion. To help maintain interest, the lecturer should remember the following key points: conciseness, simplicity, eye contact, variations in speed and volume of speech, and the use of personal experience and questions (Mackway-Jones and Walker, 1999).

Skill sessions

As resuscitation involves essentially practical skills, it is important to ensure that any training session allocates plenty of time for these skills to

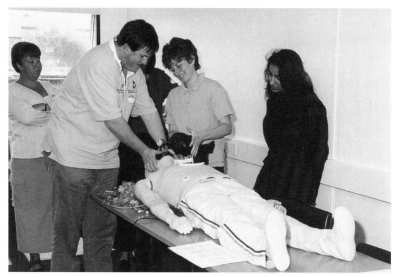

Figure 12.1 Skill session

be taught and practised. Skill sessions provide an opportunity to learn a skill and to debate relevant issues (Figure 12.1). They should be put into the context of the resuscitation procedure, and be undertaken in small groups (ideally four to six persons). They should take into account the prior experience and knowledge of the students, and build on this.

Shared aspects of teaching, learning and prior experience will promote both positive regard and mutual respect. Positive feedback, encouragement and guidance are also particularly important when teaching practical skills.

Mackway-Jones and Walker (1999) suggests a four-stage approach for teaching a practical skill.

Four-stage approach for teaching a practical skill

1. The instructor demonstrates the skill silently (silent run-through). The skill is carried out at normal speed without explanation and commentary, except what would normally be said in the clinical situation. This allows the student to observe the procedure carefully without distraction.
2. The instructor demonstrates the skill again, but this time with a commentary. It will be broken down into small steps, and will generally not be at normal speed.
3. The student provides the commentary while the instructor demonstrates the skill. This stage is used because a skill is more likely to be learned if the student can describe it in detail (Mackway-Jones and Walker, 1999). If the student is hesitant, the instructor can prompt by leading with the actions. On the other hand, confident candidates can describe the different stages of the skill before they are demonstrated. Any errors must be corrected immediately.
4. The student demonstrates the skill together with a commentary. Each student then talks through and demonstrates the skill. The instructor now has an opportunity to observe each student and ensure that he or she has understood and is competent at the skill.

Simulated cardiac arrest scenarios

Simulated cardiac arrest scenarios are a further method of teaching resuscitation skills (Figure 12.2). They can help to develop teamwork and place the subject of maternal resuscitation into context. They are a particularly useful method of training, because maternal cardiac arrests are so rare.

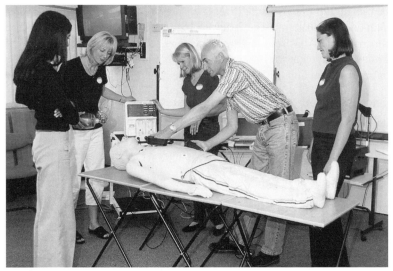

Figure 12.2   Simulated cardiac arrest scenario

The scenarios should form a major part of any training session, and they follow on logically from the teaching and practice of individual skills (e.g. bag/valve/mask resuscitation and chest compressions). They are a way of 'putting it all together' in a systematic and meaningful way. There are many advantages to this form of training:

- it is ideal for training in the clinical area
- it can help to evaluate both an individual and a group performance (Kaye *et al.*, 1986)
- it allows practitioners to practise their skills and to work as a team managing a 'cardiac arrest'
- it can help to bridge the theory/practice gap
- it can increase efficiency and credibility, improve communication and decision making, and reduce anxiety (Wynne *et al.*, 1999).

National courses

The Management of Obstetric Emergencies and Trauma course

This is a 2-day course aimed at registrars and senior clinicians in obstetrics and anaesthetics. It is designed to update clinical skills in maternal resuscitation and obstetric emergencies. Each topic is introduced by a short summary lecture, which is followed by skills practice based on real life scenarios. Midwives are encouraged to attend as observers. For further information, telephone 01782 554656.

The Advanced Life Support in Obstetrics course

The Advanced Life Support in Obstetrics (ALSO) Course was developed in the USA and imported to the UK to improve the training in obstetric emergency management. It is a skill-enhancing course modelled on other advanced life support courses. Practitioners who have attended the course have reported a significant increase in their level of perceived competence in the management of obstetric emergencies (Beasley *et al.*, 1994). For further information, telephone 0191 276 5738.

Obstetric Emergencies course

The Obstetric Emergencies course, which has been set up at the Manor Hospital in Walsall, is mainly a practical course aimed at junior medical staff just starting work in obstetrics. Both theoretical and practical aspects of maternal resuscitation are covered, as well as other obstetric emergencies. For further information, contact the Resuscitation Training Department on 01922 656575.

Resuscitation Council (UK) Advanced Life Support course

The Advanced Life Support (ALS) course is designed to teach the theory and practical skills required to manage a cardiac arrest in adults from the time when the arrest seems imminent until the patient is transferred to an intensive care department or dies.

The course is run over a minimum of 2 days, and comprises lectures, practical sessions, scenarios and assessments. A course manual is forwarded to the participants approximately 4 weeks prior to the start of the course. For further information, contact the Resuscitation Council UK (tel. 020 7388 4678).

Delivery Suite Emergencies Course

This course has been set up at the Manor Hospital in Walsall. It is a one-day course aimed at midwives. The emphasis is on practical hands-on refresher training. For further information, contact the Resuscitation Training Department on 01922 656367.

Evaluation of resuscitation training/courses

All courses and training sessions should be continually evaluated to determine whether learning objectives are being met and whether the teaching format is appropriate. In addition, it is beneficial to audit resuscitation skills and decision making in the clinical area using realistic scenarios. This method of audit will not only identify any educational requirements, but will also highlight any problems with the resuscitation equipment and procedures. It is the view of the authors that undertaking maternal resuscitation scenarios in the clinical area (e.g. the delivery suite) is an excellent method of audit, and should form an integral part of all maternal resuscitation training programmes.

Training manikins/models

Recent technological advances have enabled the manufacture of life-like training manikins and models. These are transforming training, because a greater number of clinical skills can now be demonstrated and practised in a controlled 'classroom' environment. A general overview of what is currently available follows.

Airway management models

There are a number of adult airway management manikins available (Figure 12.3). Most are anatomically correct in size and detail and benefit from having realistic landmarks, including nostrils, tongue, oro- and nasopharynx, larynx, epiglottis, vocal cords, trachea, oesophagus, inflatable lungs and stomach.

Airway management skills that can be demonstrated and practised include the sizing and insertion of the oropharyngeal airway (Guedel airway), suction and intubation. However, it is not possible realistically to perform facemask ventilation on some manikins, because the maintenance of an open airway is not always necessary to achieve chest rise. An adult manikin is the better alternative.

Resuscitation manikins

Both basic and advanced full-sized manikins are now available. Most basic ones can provide detailed and 'real time' feedback. The Skill Meter Resusci-Anne can provide a post-training evaluation, quantifying correct

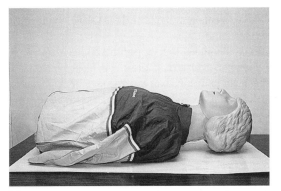

(a)

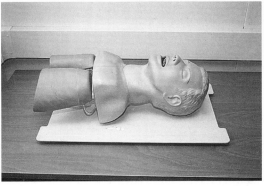

(b)

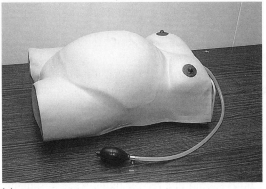

(c)

Figure 12.3 Training manikins and models

performance in percentages. It can also provide compression rates and ventilation/compression ratios.

Multifunctional advanced life support manikins are ideal for training in team management of a maternal arrest. Features generally include ECG monitoring, basic and advanced airway management (including intubation, defibrillation, cannulation and drug administration) and, of course, basic life support. One even vomits! Practitioners can undertake tasks concurrently, providing a more realistic and interactive training session.

Useful addresses

Training manikins are available from a number of companies, including:

Laerdal Medical
Laerdal House
Goodmeade Road
Orpington
Kent BR6 0HX
(Tel. 01689 876634)

Medtronic Physio-Control
Leamington Court
Andover House
Newfound
Basingstoke
Hampshire RG23 7HE
(Tel. 01256 782727)

Timesco of London
Timesco House
1 Knights Road
London E16 2AT
(Tel. 020 7511 1234)

Summary

The importance of resuscitation training has been discussed in this chapter. Retention of skills is poor, and regular training and re-training are required to ensure that competence and skills are maintained at a satisfactory level.

Appendix

Procedure for insertion of the laryngeal mask airway

The following procedure for insertion of a laryngeal mask airway (LMA) (Figure A1) is based on recommendations from the European Resuscitation Council (1998).

1. Select an appropriate sized LMA and ensure that the cuff is completely deflated.
2. Lubricate the outer cuff (i.e. the part that will not be in contact with the larynx).
3. Ensure that the casualty is in a supine position with the head and neck in alignment. If possible, slightly extend the head (**NB:** only when cervical spine injury is not suspected).

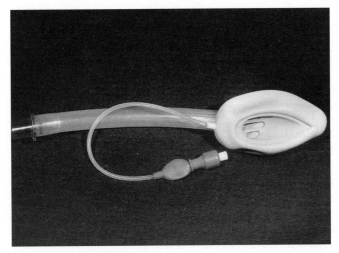

Figure A1 Laryngeal mask airway

4. Hold the tube like a pen and introduce the LMA into the mouth with the distal aperture facing the feet of the casualty. This can be undertaken either from behind the casualty or, if this is not possible, from the front.

5. Advance the tip, while applying the tip to the surface of the palate, until it reaches the wall of the posterior pharynx.

6. Push the mask backwards and downwards until it reaches the back of the hypopharynx and resistance is felt. The black line on the tube should be aligned with the nasal septum.

7. Inflate the cuff with the specified amount of air. If the position is correct, the tube will lift out of the mouth slightly (1–2 cm) and the larynx is pushed forward.

8. Confirm the LMA placement by auscultating the chest during inflation, and observe for bilateral chest movement. A small air leak is acceptable, although a large one would suggest malposition.

9. Insert a biteblock or oropharyngeal airway, and secure the LMA with a 3-cm bandage.

Bibliography

Adams, S., Whitlock, M., Higgs, R. *et al.* (1994). Should relatives be allowed to watch resuscitation? *Br. Med. J.*, **308**, 1687–9.

Aitkenhead, A. R. (1991). Drug administration during CPR: what route? *Resuscitation*, **22**, 191–5.

Archer, G. W. and Marx, G. F. (1974). Arterial oxygen tension during apnoea in parturient women. *Br. J. Anaesth.*, **46**, 358.

Bahr, J., Klingler, H., Panzer, W. *et al.* (1997). Skills of lay people in checking the carotid pulse. *Resuscitation*, **35**, 23–6.

Barron, W. M. (1984). The pregnant surgical patient: medical evaluation and management. *Ann. Int. Med.*, **101**, 683–91.

Baskett, P., Nolan, J. and Parr, M. (1996). Tidal volumes which are perceived to be adequate for resuscitation. *Resuscitation*, **3**, 231–4.

Beasley, J. W., Damos, J. R., Roberts, R. G. *et al.* (1994). The Advanced Life Support in Obstetrics Course. A national program to enhance obstetric emergency skills and to support maternity care practice. *Arch. Fam. Med.*, **3(12)**, 1037–41.

Bieniarz, J., Crottogini, J. J., Curuchet, E. *et al.* (1968). Autoclaval compression by the uterus in late human pregnancy. *Am. J. Obstet. Gynecol.*, **100**, 203.

British Association of A & E Medicine and Royal College of Nursing (1994). *Bereavement Care in A & E Departments*. RCN.

British Medical Association and Royal Pharmaceutical Society of Great Britain (1999). *British National Formulary*. BMA.

British Medical Association, Resuscitation Council UK, Royal College of Nursing (1999). *Decisions relating to cardiopulmonary resuscitation. A joint statement from the British Medical Association, the Resuscitation Council UK and the Royal College of Nursing*, BMA, London.

Bury Medical Audit (1994). *Audit of the Care of Bereaved Relatives following Sudden Death*. 121 Silver Street, Bury BL9 0EN.

Bussen, S., Schwarzmann, G. and Steck, T. (1997). Clinical aspects of amniotic fluid embolism. Illustration based on a case report (in German). *Zeit. Geburts. Neonatol.*, **201(3)**, 95–8.

Chalk, A. (1995). Should relatives be present in the resuscitation room? *J. A&E Nursing*, **3(2)**, 58–61.

Clark, S. L., Cotton, D. B. and Lee, W. (1989). Central hemodynamic assessment of the normal term pregnancy. *Am. J. Obstet. Gynecol.*, **161**, 1439.

Cobbe, S., Redmond, M., Watson, J. *et al.* (1991). "Heartstart Scotland" – initial experience of a national scheme for out-of-hospital defibrillation. *British Medical Journal*, **302**, 1517–20.

Cox, C. and Grady, K. (1999). *Managing Obstetric Emergencies*. BIOS.

Curry, J. J. and Quintana, F. J. (1970). Myocardial infarction with ventricular fibrillation during pregnancy treated by direct current defibrillation with fetal survival. *Chest*, **58**, 82.

Department of Health (1993). *Confidential Enquiries into Maternal Deaths in the United Kingdom 1988–1990*. HMSO.

Department of Health (1996). *Immunisation against Infectious Disease*. HMSO, London.

Department of Health (1998). *Why Mothers Die: Report on Confidential Enquiries into Maternal Deaths in the United Kingdom 1994–1996*. HMSO.

Dildy, G. A. and Clarke, S. L. (1995). Cardiac arrest during pregnancy. *Obst. Gynecol. Clin. North Am.*, **22(2)**, 304–14.

Dimond, B. (1994). *The Legal Aspects of Midwifery*. Books for Midwives, Hale.

Doan-Wiggins, L. (1996). Resuscitation of the pregnant patient suffering sudden death in cardiac arrest. In: *The Science and Practice of Resuscitation Medicine*, pp. 812–19. Williams & Wilkins.

Dorian, P., Fain, E. S., Davy, J. M. *et al.* (1986). Lidocaine causes a reversible, concentration-dependent increase in defibrillation energy requirements. *J. Am. Coll. Cardiol.*, **8**, 327–32.

Drife, J. (1997). Management of primary postpartum haemorrhage. *Br. J. Obstet. Gynaecol.*, **104**, 275–7.

Eberle, B., Dick, W. F., Schneider, T. *et al.* (1996). Checking the carotid pulse check: diagnostic accuracy of first responders in patients with and without a pulse. *Resuscitation*, **33**, 107–16.

Emerman, C.L., Bellon, E. M., Lukens, T. W. *et al.* (1990). The effect of bolus injection on circulation times during cardiac arrest. *Am. J. Emerg. Med.*, **8**, 190–93.

European Resuscitation Council (1998). *European Resuscitation Council Guidelines for Resuscitation*. Elsevier.

Ewan, P. W. (1996). Clinical study of peanut and nut allergy in 62 consecutive patients; new features and associations. *Br. Med. J.*, **312**, 1074–8.

Fisher, M. (1986). Clinical observations on the pathophysiology and treatment of anaphylactic cardiovascular collapse. *Anaesth. Intensive Care*, **14**, 17–21.

Fisher, M. (1995). Treatment of acute anaphylaxis. *British Medical Journal*, **311**, 731–3.

Flesche, C. W., Brewer, S., Mandel, L. P. *et al.* (1994). The ability of health professionals to check the carotid pulse. *Circulation*, **90**, 1–288.

Goodwin, A. P. L. and Pearce, A. J. (1992). The human wedge. *Anaesthesia*, **47**, 433–4.

Greer, I. (1997). Thrombo-embolic disease in obstetrics and gynaecology. *Clin. Obstet. Gynaecol.*, **2**, 403–615.

Guildner, C. (1976) Resuscitation – opening the airway: a comparative study of techniques for opening the airway obstructed by the tongue. *J. Am. Coll. Emerg. Phys.*, **5**, 588–90.

Hapnes, S. A. and Robertson, C. E. (1992). CPR – drug delivery routes and systems. *Resuscitation*, **24**, 137–42.

Harrison, R. and Maull, K. (1982). Pocket mask ventilation: a superior method of acute airway management. *Ann. Emerg. Med.*, **11**, 74–76.

Henderson, C. and Jones, K. (Eds) (1996). *Essential Midwifery*. Mosby, London.

Hess, D. and Baran, C. (1985). Ventilatory volumes using mouth-to-mouth, mouth-to-mask and bag-valve-mask techniques. *Am. J. Emerg. Med.*, **3**, 292–6.

Hwang, J., Chuang, H., Wei, T. and Yang, Y. (1993). Successful resuscitation of amniotic fluid embolism during Caesarean section: a case report. *Ma Tsui Hsueh Tsa Chi Anaesthesiologica Sinica*, **31(3)**, 191–4.

Idris, A., Florete, O., Melker, R. and Chandra, N. (1996). *Physiology of ventilation, oxygenation and carbon dioxide elimination during cardiac arrest.* In: *Cardiac Arrest: The Science and Practice of Resuscitation Medicine*, Paradis, N., Halperin, H., Nowak, R. (Eds). Williams & Wilkins, London.

Ilsaas, C., Husby, C., Koller, M. *et al.* (1998). Cardiac arrest due to massive pulmonary embolism following Caesarean section, successful resuscitation and pulmonary embolectomy. *Acta Anaesthesiol. Scand.*, **42(2)**, 264–6.

Jesudian, M., Harrison, R., Keenan, R. and Maull, K. (1985). Bag-valve-mask ventilation; two rescuers are better than one: preliminary report. *Crit. Care. Med.*, **13**, 122–3.

Jevon, P. (2000). Anaphylaxis. *Emergency Management*, **96(14)**, 39–40.

Jowett, N. and Thompson, D. R. (1995). *Comprehensive Coronary Care*, 2nd edn. Scutari Press.

Kaye, W. and Mancini, M. (1986). Use of Mega Code to evaluate team leader performance during advanced cardiac life support. *Critical Care Medicine*, **14(2)**, 99–104.

Katz, V. L., Dotters, D. J. and Droegemueller, W. (1986). Perimortem Caesarean delivery. *Obstet. Gynecol.*, **68**, 571.

Kerr, M. G. (1965). The mechanical effects of the gravid uterus in late pregnancy. *J. Obstet. Gynaecol. Br. Comm.*, **72**, 513.

Khun, G. J., White, B. C. and Swetnam, R. E. (1981). Peripheral vs central circulation times during CPR: a pilot study. *Ann. Emerg. Med.*, **10**, 417–19.

Killam, A. (1985). Amniotic fluid embolism. *Clin. Obstet. Gynecol.*, **28**, 32–6.

Lattuada, H. P. (1952). Postmortem Caesarean section. *Am. J. Surg.*, **84**, 212.

Lau, G. (1994). A case of sudden maternal death associated with resuscitative liver injury. *Forensic Sci. Int.*, **67(2)**, 127–32.

Lawrence, P. and Sivaneswaran, N. (1985). Ventilation during cardiopulmonary resuscitation: which method? *Med. J. Austr.*, **143**, 443–6.

Lee, W. and Cotton, D. B. (1991). Cardiorespiratory changes during pregnancy. In: *Critical Care Obstetrics*, 2nd edn (S. L. Clark, D. B. Cotton, J. D. Hankins *et al.*, eds), pp. 75. Blackwell Scientific Publications.

Lee, R., Rodgers, B., White, L. and Harvey, R. (1986). Cardiopulmonary resuscitation of pregnant women. *Am. J. Med.*, **81**, 311.

Leitner, L., Bauer, P. and Fabsits, M. (1995). Amniotic fluid embolism – a case report with positive outcome (in German). *Anasthesiol. Intensivmed. Schmerzther.*, **30(2)**, 113–15.

Lopez-Zeno, J. A., Carlo, W. A., O'Grady, J. P. *et al.* (1990). Infant survival following delayed postmortem Caesarean delivery. *Obstet. Gynecol.*, **76**, 991–2.

Lowenstein, S., Libby, L., Mountain, R., *et al.* (1981). Cardiopulmonary resuscitation by medical and surgical house officer. *Lancet*, **2**, 679.

Mace, S. E. (1990). Differences in plasma lidocaine levels with endotracheal drug therapy secondary to total volume of fluid administered. *Resuscitation*, **20**, 185–91.

Mackway-Jones, K. and Walker, M. (1999). *Pocket Guide to Teaching for Medical Instructors.* BMJ Books, London.

Mander, R. (1994). *Loss and Bereavement in Childbearing*, 1st edn. Blackwell Science.

Mantel, G., Buchmann, E., Rees, H. *et al.* (1998). Severe acute maternal morbidity: a pilot study of a definition of a near miss. *Br. J. Obstet. Gynaecol.*, **105**, 985–90.

McKenna, S. and Glendon, A. (1985). Occupational first aid training: decay in cardiopulmonary resuscitation (CPR) skills. *J. Occ. Psychology*, **58**, 109–17.

Mehta, S. (1990). A supraglottic oropharyngeal airway. *Anaesthesia*, **45**, 893–4.

Melker, R. J. (1985). Recommendations for ventilation during cardiopulmonary resuscitation: a time for change? *Crit. Care Med.*, **13(2)**, 882–3.

Melker, R. J. and Banner, M. J. (1985). Ventilation during CPR: two rescuer standards re-appraised. *Ann. Emerg. Med.*, **14**, 197.

Michael, J. R., Guerci, A. D., Koeler, R. C. *et al.* (1984). Mechanisms by which epinephrine augments cerebral and myocardial perfusion during cardiopulmonary resuscitation in dogs. *Circulation*, **69**, 822–35.

Morgam, M. (1979). Amniotic fluid embolism: review. *Anaesthesia*, **34**, 20–32.

Morris, S. and Willis, B. A. (1999). Resuscitation in pregnancy. In: *ABC of Resuscitation*, 4th edn, pp. 31–4. BMJ Publishing.

Muzzi, D., Losasso, T. and Cucchiara, R. (1991). Complications of a nasopharyngeal airway in a patient with a basilar skull fracture. *Anaesthesiology*, **74**, 366–8.

Myint, Y., Bailey, P. and Milne, B. (1992). Cardiorespiratory arrest following combined spinal epidural anaesthesia for Caesarean section. *Anaesthesia*, **48(8)**, 684–6.

Noble, W. (1997). *Confidential Enquiries into Maternal Deaths in the United Kingdom: West Midlands Region Guidance for Health Professionals.* West Midlands NHS Executive.

Nolan, J. and Gwinnett, C. (1998). 1998 European guidelines on resuscitation. *Br. Med. J.*, **316**, 1844–5.

Owens, M., Robertson, P., Twomey, C. *et al.* (1995). The incidence of gastroesophageal reflux using the laryngeal mask: a comparison with the face mask using esophageal lumen pH electrodes. *Anaes. Analg.*, **80**, 980–4.

Pagan-Carlo, L., Spencer, K., Robertson, C. *et al.* (1996). Transthoracic defibrillation: importance of avoiding electrode placement directly on the female breast. *J. Am. Coll. Cardiol.*, **27**, 449–52.

Patel, L., Radivan, F. S. and David, T. J. (1994). Management of anaphylactic reactions to food. *Arch. Dis. Child*, **71**, 370–75.

Project Team of the Resuscitation Council (UK) (1999). The emergency medical treatment of anaphylactic reactions. *J. A & E Med.*, **16(4)**, 243–7.

Rees, G. A. D. and Willis, B. A. (1988). Resuscitation in late pregnancy. *Anaesthesia*, **43**, 347–9.

Renner, S. (1991). I desperately wanted to see my son. *Br. Med. J.*, **302**, 356.

Resuscitation Council UK (2000). *Advanced Life Support Manual*, 4th edn. Resuscitation Council UK.

Royal College of Obstetricians and Gynaecologists Working Party (1995). *Risk Assessment Profile for Thromboembolism in Caesarean Section. Report of a*

Working Party on Prophylaxis against Thromboembolism in Gynaecology and Obstetrics. RCOG.

Royal College of Physicians (1987). *Resuscitation from cardiopulmonary arrest: training and organisation.* Royal College of Physicians, London.

Safar, P. (1958). Ventilatory efficacy of mouth-to-mouth artificial respiration: airway obstruction during manual and mouth-to-mouth artificial ventilation. *JAMA*, **67**, 341.

Satin, A. J. and Hankins, J. D. (1991). Cardiopulmonary resuscitation in pregnancy. In: *Critical Care Obstetrics*, 2nd edn (S. L. Clark, D. B. Cotton, J. D. Hankins *et al.*, eds). Blackwell Scientific Publications.

Schierhout, G. and Roberts, I. (1998). Fluid resuscitation with colloid or crystalloid solutions in critically ill patients: a systematic review of randomised trials. *Br. Med. J.*, **316**, 961–4.

Schilling, R. (1994). Should relatives watch resuscitation? *Br. Med. J.*, **309**, 406.

Sedgwick, M., Dalziel, K., Watson, J. *et al.* (1994). The causative rhythm in out-of-hospital cardiac arrests witnessed by the emergency medical services in the Heartstart Scotland project. *Resuscitation*, **27**, 55–9.

Seldon, B. S. and Burke, T. J. (1988). Complete maternal and fetal recovery after prolonged cardiac arrest. *Ann. Emerg. Med.*, **17**, 346.

Sellick, B. A. (1961). Cricoid pressure to control regurgitation of stomach contents during the induction of anaesthesia. *Lancet*, **2**, 404.

Simons, F. E., Roberts, J. R., Gu, X. *et al.* (1998). Epinephrine absorption in children with a history of anaphylaxis. *J. Allergy Clin. Immunol.*, **101**, 33–7.

Sirna, S. J., Ferguson, D. W., Charbonnier, F. *et al.* (1988). Factors affecting transthoracic impedance during electrical cardioversion. *Am. J. Cardiol.*, **62**, 1048–52.

Skinner, D. and Vincent, R. (1993) *Cardiopulmonary Resuscitation.* Oxford University Press, Oxford, UK.

Smith, S. and Hatchett, R. (1992) Perceived competence in cardiopulmonary resuscitation, knowledge and skills among 50 qualified nurses. *Intensive and Critical Care Nursing*, **8**, 76–81.

Steedman, D. J. and Robertson, C. E. (1992). Acid–base changes in arterial and central venous blood during cardiopulmonary resuscitation. *Arch. Emerg. Med.*, **9**, 169–76.

Stokes, I. M., Evans, J. and Stone, M. (1984). Myocardial infarction and cardiac arrest in the second trimester followed by assisted vaginal delivery under epidural analgesia at 38 weeks' gestation: case report. *Br. J. Obstet. Gynaecol.*, **91**, 197.

Strong, T. H. and Lowe, R. A. (1989). *Perimortem Caesarean section.* J. Emerg. Med., **7**, 489.

Sullivan, J. M. and Ramanathan, K. B. (1985). Management of medical problems in pregnancy: severe cardiac disease. *N. Engl. J. Med.*, **313**, 304.

Swartjes, J., Schutte, M. and Bleker, O. (1992). Management of eclampsia: cardiopulmonary arrest resulting from magnesium sulfate overdose. *Eur. J. Obstet., Gynecol. Reprod. Biol.*, **47(1)**, 73–5.

Taylor, G. J., Tucker, W. M. and Greene, H. L. (1977). Importance of prolonged compression during cardiopulmonary resuscitation in man. *N. Engl. J. Med.*, **296**, 1515–17.

Tunstall-Pedoe, H., Bailey, L., Chamberlain, D. *et al.* (1992). Survey of 3765 cardiopulmonary resuscitations in British Hospitals (the BRESUS study). *British Medical Journal*, **304**, 1347–51.

UKCC (1998a). *Guidelines for Records and Record Keeping*. UKCC, London.

UKCC (1998b). *Midwives Rules and Code of Practice*. UKCC, London.

Windle, W. F. (1968). Brain damage at birth: functional and structural modifications with time. *J. Am. Med. Assoc.*, **206,** 1967.

Wright, B. (1996). *Sudden Death, A Research Base for Practice*, 2nd edn. Churchill Livingstone.

Wynne, G., Marteau, T., Johnson, M. *et al.* (1987). Inability of trained nurses to perform basic life support. *British Medical Journal*, **294**, 1198–9.

Wynne, G., Gwinnutt, C., Bingham, R. *et al.* (1999). *Teaching Resuscitation.* In: *ABC of Resuscitation*, Colquhoun, M., Handley, A., Evans, T. (Eds). BMJ Books, London.

Zoltie, N., Sloan, J. and Wright, B. (1994). Observed resuscitation may affect a doctor's performance. *Br. Med. J.*, **309, **406.

Index

Acidosis, 67
Acute Respiratory Distress Syndrome
   (ARDS), 6
Adrenaline:
   anaphylaxis, 74
      self-administration, 74
   resuscitation, 13, 66
Advance directives, 97
Advanced life support, 54–69
   drugs, 66–8
   post-resuscitation care, 69
   Resuscitation Council Algorithm, 55–59
   training courses, 107
Airedale Hospital NHS Trust v Bland,
   94–5
Airway:
   clearing, 39
   laryngeal mask, 42, 111–12
   models, 108
   nasopharyngeal, 41
   opening, 37, 38–39
      in trauma, 39
   oropharyngeal, 39–1
Alkalosis, 13
ALSO course, 107
Amniotic fluid embolism, 6–7, 63
   register, 80
Anaesthesia, 7, 64
Anapen®, 74
Anaphylaxis, 70–6
   causes, 71
   clinical presentation, 72
   defined, 71
   diagnosis, 72
   follow-up, 76
   management, 72–6
   pathogenesis, 71
Anatomical changes in pregnancy, 10–16
Antepartum haemorrhage, 6
Antepartum pulmonary embolism, 3
Anti-arrhythmics, 58
Antihistamines, 75
Aortocaval compression, 13, 14

Arrhythmias, 32–4, 56, 57
Asystole, 32–33, 57, 58
   following defibrillation, 58–59
Atropine, 27, 58, 66
   dose, 66–7
Audit, 98, 99, 108
Automatic external defibrillation, 61, 62

Baby, see Fetus
Bad news, breaking to relatives, 89–90
   over the telephone, 90–1
Bag/valve/mask ventilation, 44–6
Basic life support, 35–53
   airway management, 37, 38–42
   chest compressions, 37, 48–52
   getting help, 37–8
   gravid uterus displacement, 48–50
   initial assessment, 36–7
   mother's position, 48–50
   ventilation, 42–7
Bereavement, 88–91
Beta blockers, 27
Blood pressure, 12
Bolam test, 94–5
Bolitho v City and Hackney Hospital, 95
Breathing checks, 37
Bupivacaine, 64

Caesarean section:
   emergency, 16, 68–69
   thromboembolism risk, 3, 4, 5
Calcium, 64, 67
Cardiac arrest, causes, 61–4
Cardiac arrest trolley, see Resuscitation
   trolley
Cardiac arrhythmias, 32–4, 56, 57
Cardiac disease, 8
Cardiac monitoring, 26–34
Cardiac output, 12, 58
Cardiac tamponade, 63
Cardiff resuscitation wedge, 49

Cardiovascular system, 10–14
Carotid pulse, 37
Central venous cannulation, 65, 66
Chest compressions, 37, 48–52
Chlorpheniramine, 75
Choking, 52
Clinical negligence, 93, 95
Colloids, 75
Community midwife's resuscitation bag, 24, 25
Complaints, 99
Compliance, 15
Confidential Enquiries into Maternal Deaths, 81, 82, 86, 87
Consent to be resuscitated, withdrawal, 97
Co-ordinators, 83
Cricoid pressure, 47–8
Crystalloids, 75

Defibrillation:
  asystole following, 58–59
  automatic external, 61, 62
  equipment checks, 23–4
  paddle position, 60
  principles, 59–60
  safety, 60
  ventricular fibrillation/tachycardia, 56, 58
Delivery suite emergency course, 107
Dentures, 39
Director of Public Health, 85, 87
'Do-not-resuscitate' orders, 96
DOPE, 65
Drugs:
  administration routes, 65–6
  for anaphylaxis, 74
  resuscitation, 66–8
Duty of care, 92–5, 98

Eclampsia, 5–6, 64, 67
Electrocardiogram (ECG), 27–34
  arrhythmias, 32–4, 56
  artefacts, 30
  baseline wandering, 30
  electrodes, 30, 24
  electromechanical dissociation, 34, 57, 58
  interference, 30
  PQRST complex, 27–8
  recording problems, 29–30
  recording technique, 29
  straight line trace, 33
Electrolyte imbalance, 63
Electromechanical dissociation, 33, 57, 58
Endobronchial drug administration, 65–6

Endocarditis, 8
Epidural anaesthesia, 7, 64
Epinephrine (adrenaline):
  anaphylaxis, 74
    self-administration, 74
  resuscitation, 13, 66
Epipen®, 74, 75
Equipment, 17–25
Ethics, 92–100

Families, *see* Relatives
Fetus:
  death, registering, 84
  hypoxia protection, 15
  survival, 15–16, 68
Fluid replacement, 75
Food allergies, 71
Functional residual capacity, 13, 15

Gastric inflation during ventilation, 46–7
Gastrointestinal tract, 11, 15
General practitioners, 87
Gravid uterus displacement, 48–50
Guedel airway, 39–41

Haemorrhage, 6, 62
Head tilt/chin lift, 38
Heart:
  conduction system, 26–7
  disease and maternal death, 8
  injection into, 66
  rate:
    counter, 28–9
    nervous control, 27
    in pregnancy, 12
Human wedge, 49–50
Hydrocortisone, 75
Hyperkalaemia, 63
Hyperventilation, 13
Hypokalaemia, 63
Hypothermia, 63
Hypovolaemia, 62
Hypoxia, 13, 15, 62
Hysterectomy, emergency, 63

Intracardiac injection, 66
Intubation, 64–5

Jaw thrust, 39

Labour induction, 7
Laryngeal mask airway, 43, 111–12
Latex allergy, 71
Lectures, 104
Legal aspects, 79, 92–100
  advance directives, 97
  clinical negligence, 93, 95
  'do-not-resuscitate' order, 96
  risk management, 98–100
  standard of care, 92–5, 98
  withdrawal of consent to be resuscitated, 97
Life support, *see* Advanced life support;
  Basic life support
Lignocaine (lidocaine), 58, 67
  dose, 67

Magnesium overdose, 64, 67
Management of Obstetric Emergencies and
  Trauma course, 106–7
Manikins, 108–10
Maternal death, 1–9
  case notes, 83
  causes, 3–9
  classification, 1–3
  *Confidential Enquiries into Maternal
    Deaths*, 81, 82, 86, 87
  co-ordinators, 83
  defined, 1, 82
  direct, 2, 3–7, 82
  family concerns, *see* Relatives
  fortuitous, 2, 9, 82
  indirect, 2, 7–8, 82
  late, 3, 9, 82
  management, 83–5
  notification, 84, 85, 87
  post-mortem, 83
  religious considerations, 84
  staff support, 84
Metabolic acidosis, 67
Metabolic disorders, 63
Metabolic rate, 13
Models and manikins, 108–10
Mouth-to-mask ventilation, 43–4
Mouth-to-mouth ventilation, 42–3

Nasopharyngeal airway, 41
Negligence, 92, 95

Obstetric Emergencies course, 107
Oropharyngeal airway, 39–41

Oxygen:
  for anaphylaxis, 72
  consumption, 13
Oxytocic drugs, 7

Panic attack, 72
Physiological changes in pregnancy, 10–16
Piriton, 75
Placenta praevia, 6
Placental abruption, 6
Pneumothorax, 63
Pocket mask, 43–4
Post-mortem, 83
Postpartum haemorrhage, 6
Postpartum pulmonary embolism, 3–4
Post-resuscitation care, 69
Practical skill training, 104–5
Pre-eclampsia, 5–6, 64, 67
Protocols, 99
Psychiatric deaths, 8
Pulmonary aspiration, 15, 47
Pulmonary embolism, 3–5, 64
  prophylaxis, 3, 5, 64
  risk factors, 4
Pulseless electrical activity, 33, 57, 58

Record keeping, 77–80, 83, 99
Relatives:
  breaking bad news to, 89–90
    over the telephone, 90–1
  meeting with consultant, 85
  presence during resuscitation, 91
  religious considerations, 84
  rooms for, 88–89
Religious considerations, 84
Residual capacity, 13, 15
Respiratory acidosis, 67
Respiratory alkalosis, 13
Respiratory system, 11, 13, 15
Resusci-Anne, 108, 110
Resuscitation Council (UK) Advanced Life
  Support course, 107
Resuscitation Council (UK) Algorithms:
  Advanced Life Support, 55–59
  Automated External Defibrillation, 62
  Basic Life Support, 36
Resuscitation trolley, 17–24
  checking, 23–4
  layout, 17–22
  restocking, 24
  seals, 23
Risk management, 98–100

Safety, 60, 100
Scenario testing, 98, 105–6
Sinus bradycardia, 30–1
Sinus node, 27
Sinus rhythm, 30, 31
Sinus tachycardia, 30, 31
Skill Meter Resusci-Anne, 108, 110
Skull fracture, airway management, 41
Sodium bicarbonate, 67–8
Spinal injury, airway management, 39
Staff:
   support, 84
   training, 101–10
Standard of care, 92–5, 98
Stroke volume, 12
Suicide, 8
Sympathetic system, 27

Telephone, breaking bad news over, 90–1
Tension pneumothorax, 63
Thoracocentesis, 63
Thromboembolism, 3–5, 63
   prophylaxis, 3, 5, 64
   risk factors, 4
Tracheal intubation, 64–5
Training, 101–110
   courses, 106–8
   importance of, 101–2
   lectures, 104

   manikins/models, 108–10
   practical sessions, 104–5
   recommendations, 102
   simulated scenario testing, 105–6
   skill retention, 102, 103
Transthoracic impedance, 59–60
Trauma, airway management, 39, 41

Uteroplacental blood flow, 12–13
Uterus displacement during resuscitation,
   48–50

Vascular resistance, 12
Venous drug administration, 65, 66
Ventilation:
   bag/valve/mask, 44–6
   failure, 42
   gastric inflation during, 46–7
   mouth-to-mask (pocket mask), 43–4
   mouth-to-mouth, 42–3
   rate and volume, 46–7
Ventricular fibrillation, 32, 33, 57
   defibrillation, 56, 58
Ventricular tachycardia, 32, 33
   defibrillation, 56, 58

Wedges, 49–50